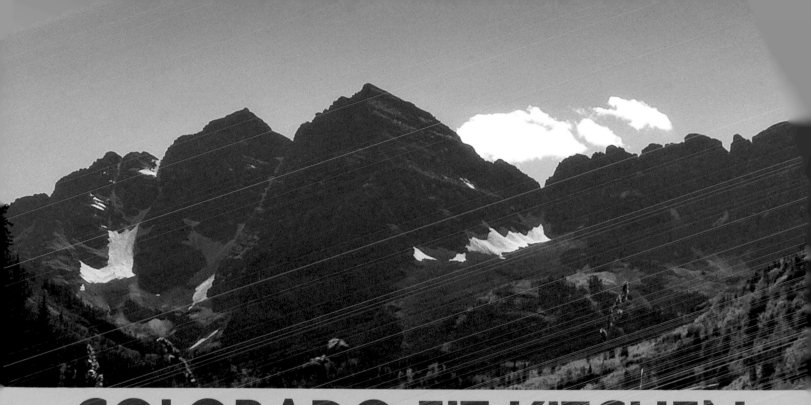

COLORADO FIT KITCHEN
Inspiring Recipes for Mind, Body, Beauty and Optimum Wellness

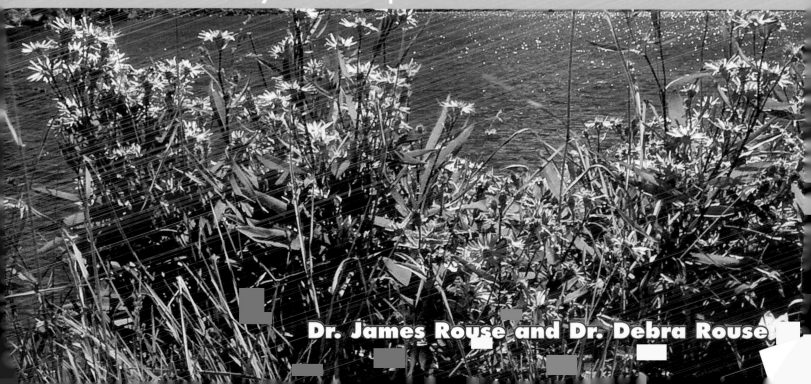

Dr. James Rouse and Dr. Debra Rouse

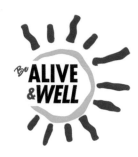

Colorado Fit Kitchen
Copyright 2010 by Be Alive & Well, LLC
Be Alive & Well, LLC
dba Optimum Wellness
PO Box 587
Indian Hills, CO 80454
303-697-6662
fax 303-697-3323
www.optimumwellness.com

Optimum Wellness is a registered dba of Be Alive & Well, LLC

Cover photo: Maroon Bells in Summer, Matthew J. Ried   www.rockylakesphoto.com.
Back Cover photos: Barn Clouds and Colorado Pond Reflection and portraits of James and Debra,
Carl Studna   www.carlstudna.com

Food photography (unless otherwise noted): Debra J. Rouse, ND
Powered Up Pasta (Butternut Squash Photo), Katie Hedrick   www.legacyzoom.com

Design & Layout by Susie Grossinger   www.susiegrossinger.com

Edited by Emily Miller, Debra Rouse, ND, and James Rouse, ND

Nutritional analysis data is calculated using MasterCook™. Calculations for the nutritional analysis in this book are based on the average number of servings listed. If two options are listed for an ingredient, the first one is used.

Information in this book is not intended to diagnose, treat, or prevent disease.

Library of Congress Control Number:
2009941481
ISBN 978-0-9843062-0-6

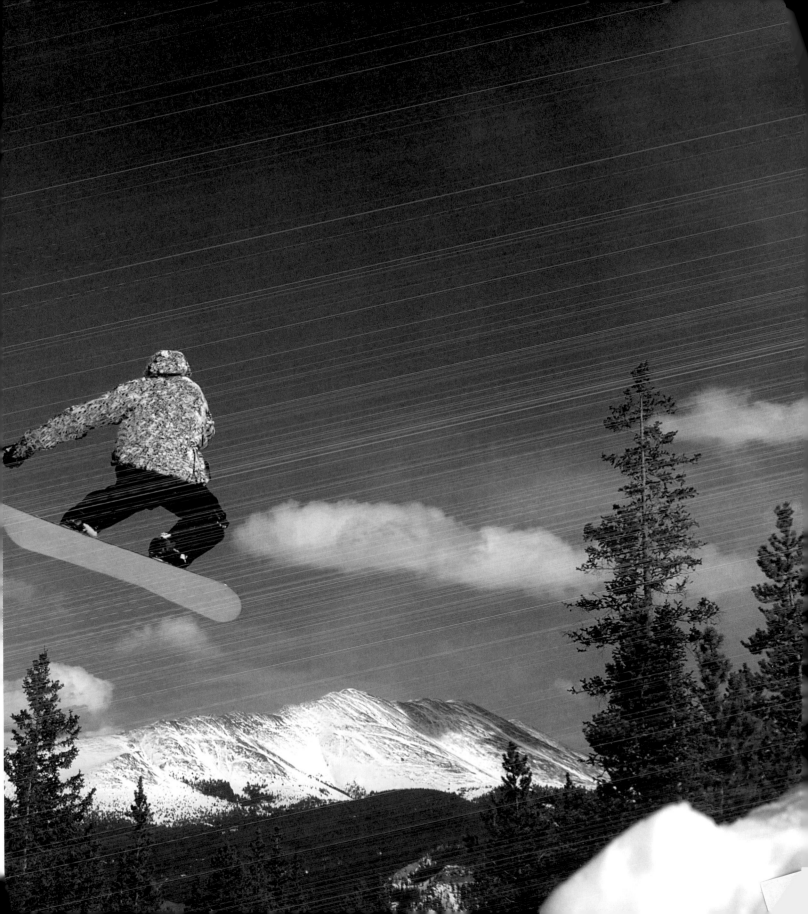

Acknowledgments:

It is quite amazing that for the most part this book came together with the work of just four of us. But that work depended on the support, love, and trust of so many incredible individuals who we would like to acknowledge here.

Susie Grossinger, our cousin, came up with the layout and design of this book. She put in long, late hours, traveled to Colorado and is just one true gem in this world.

Emily Miller, our assistant on every level and all around amazing presence. This project would've taken at least another full year had we not had your input, your editing, your test cooking and your positive Spirit and constant encouragement.

Carl Studna, photographer extraordinaire, who stepped up and said I want to take your picture for the book. You are an amazing and gifted artist. Thank you.

Carl and Cynthia, our Master Mind partners, have held this vision with us since day 1. We are so grateful.

Roger and Erica, dear friends and mentors who also held the vision and cheered us on at every step.

Dan and Lisa Sims, dear friends and true visionaries sharing the message of Optimum Wellness.

Our families who have always believed in us, we love you very much.

My partners at mix1 – you guys are the dream team – thank you!

The team at QVC, a special thank you.

John Allen and Scott Takeda have given over a decade of creative energy to Optimum Wellness. Thank you.

Mark Koebrich and Kim Christiansen at 9News, you have always been so supportive of this mission. Thank you.

Susan McNamee, friend, believer, and champion of Optimum Wellness. Thank you.

And for so many of our friends, we are grateful. This just wouldn't happen without the tribe: Ken and Lisa, Sue and Mark, Cindy, Christina and Kim, Tom and Dawn, Rita and George, Mary and Ed, Seth and Stacy, Melody and Joe, Janyn and Tom, Traci and Steve, Julie, and to all who share similar passions of food, friends, family, and God – thank you!

Dedication

With deep love and gratitude we honor our parents and daughters with the dedication of this book.

Deb:
In memory of my dad, Freddie, a wonderful health nut, who inspired in me the love of all things sweet. I love and miss you everyday.

To my mom, Nanon, who showed me how busy moms can do it all and still put a real meal on the table every night. You will always be Supermom to me, I love you.

James:
In memory of my dad, Bucky, although we did not share a love of healthy food, we did share the love of persistence and purpose, both of which made this book possible — thanks for the life lessons Dad.

To my mom, Carol, whose love of family, friends, and dinner parties has always been an inspiration to me, thanks Mom. I love you.

And for our two beautiful angels, Dakota and Elli, who have been a part of this amazing journey all along.

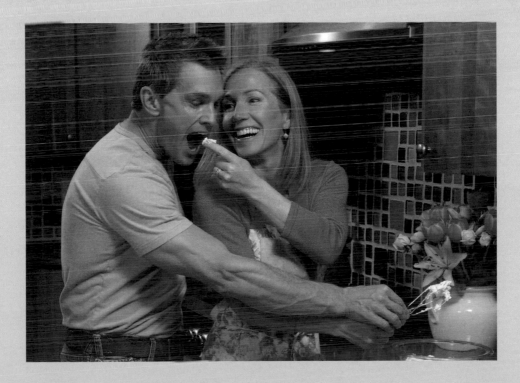

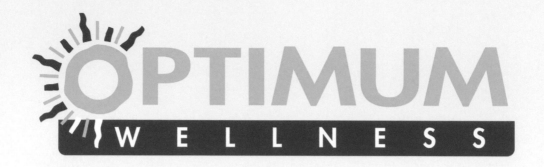

Introduction – Why We Decided to Write a Cookbook

Our love affair with natural foods blossomed nearly 20 years ago when we were beginning our naturopathic medical education in Portland, Oregon. We started medical school, fell in love, opened the Common Sense Cafe with a few friends to help pay for books, and put our love of food to work turning people on to the power and benefit of healthy, clean eating.

After graduation we began seeing patients in New Mexico and Colorado. No matter whom we saw or treated, we always spoke about the importance of healthy eating. We often suggested ways to "sneak" healthy ingredients into menus and meal plans, encouraging our patients to see food as the necessary foundation for building a life of inspired well-being, balanced energy, a beautiful body, radiant skin and optimism.

The one-on-one connections we made in private practice stirred a desire in us to want to reach even more people, beyond our clinic walls. We dreamed of ways we could touch, serve and inspire an even broader audience outside of our clinic walls. In 1999 the Columbine High School shooting tragedy occurred, urging us to make more of a contribution and commitment to bringing a message of optimism to the community. Our intention was to set a stage for healing by bringing our wellness philosophy to the greater Denver Metro area.

Although neither of us had any real experience with television, James approached the local NBC affiliate, KUSA (9News), in Denver and lobbied hard for over a year for a chance to do a segment on wellness and healthy eating. Finally we received the "yes" and launched Optimum Wellness and The Fit Kitchen.

The Fit Kitchen was a twice-weekly cooking segment on the afternoon news. The news anchors were encouraging, loving, occasionally skeptical but always game for good food. Many of the recipes in the cookbook came out of the Fit Kitchen. The Colorado Fit Kitchen makes healthy cooking do-able and delicious.

Food is powerful medicine. The relationship between a healthy, balanced, whole foods diet and disease prevention is well documented. Our recipes take the guesswork out of how to put it all together. We believe that the most effective approach to eating well is not only utilizing healthy ingredients but also making it simple, fun and exciting to prepare food. Most importantly it must taste great. We have always enjoyed hearing "are you sure this is healthy?" Or, "this can't be good for me!" This is music to our ears and we love that our patients, viewers, customers, friends and family alike always love what we are cooking!

What is our food philosophy? We consider ourselves conscious omnivores – we love all kinds of food that has been conscientiously grown and raised. We are about keeping it real, keeping it clean and natural. We are a bit over-zealous when it comes to being sure that there are no fake ingredients, no artificial colors, preservatives, and no ingredients that you cannot pronounce! We choose ingredients that offer many health benefits; ones that are naturally rich in antioxidants to further support your well-being, prevent disease and premature aging. The calories and portions are the right size and because they are balanced and rich in fiber your satisfaction and fulfillment will be magnified. We know that when you eat well, when you feed your mind and body with the right kinds of foods, your metabolism will run impeccably, your mind will be clear with intention and focus, your attitude and outlook optimistic and abundant. Simply, when you eat our meals, snacks and entrees, you are going to be living, looking and feeling your best.

Our love of great tasting and vital food has been a blessing in so many ways. It has helped nourish our two daughters, build successful lifestyle-based medical practices, and has been the cornerstone of Optimum Wellness Media (now 10 years old). Optimum Wellness media consists of our television spots, our bi-monthly Optimum Wellness magazine, and our website, www.optimumwellness.com. This is where we introduce viewers and readers to healthy lifestyle practices, organics and inspired whole food recipes, and other motivational and inspirational messages of encouragement and possibility.

And one more thing you should know about us, we have always loved to exercise. Exercise and healthy eating are meant to go together. We both continue to train for triathlons, marathons and life. In 2006, James co-founded a functional beverage company called mix1 (www.mix1life.com) to address and support the nutrition and performance needs of life athletes and elite athletes nationally. We love mix1 because not only is it an amazing beverage for athletes, but it is the perfect grab and go breakfast or between meals snack for everyday folks who are looking to keep their minds and bodies balanced and energized at all times. We may mention mix1 once or twice in the book – it makes especially tasty popsicles!

You may wonder if there any "side effects" of eating with us. Yes, you may experience many positive side effects including better overall energy and clarity, quality sleep, less anxiety, clearer more radiant skin, less sugar cravings and quite possibly an uncontrollable urge to share this cookbook, its recipes and philosophy with friends, family and total strangers. We are fully supportive of honoring that urge!

There are just a few table rules for you to follow:

- Be open to discovery. There is no such thing as being perfect in your Fit Kitchen. Have fun – play with the recipes, experiment and make them your own. It's all good!

- Embrace preparation and cooking as part of the experience not just as a means to an end...eating. Learn to love the act and practice of being in your kitchen and see it as a place where your inner artist, child and chef show up and play.

- Always remember that diet comes from the Latin word diaeta, which means, "way of life." Celebrate eating well, use food as a means to raise your vitality along with your joy.

Our wish is that you are open to using these recipes and our food philosophy as part of your own vision to create and sustain Optimum Wellness for you and your loved ones. We believe that every moment of your life you are blessed with the power to choose how you wish to show up in the world and choose to be of service and be a beneficial presence. Ultimately a great way to be is to love, serve, share and inspire. We believe this is the best recipe for life. Enjoy and be well!

~James and Debra Rouse

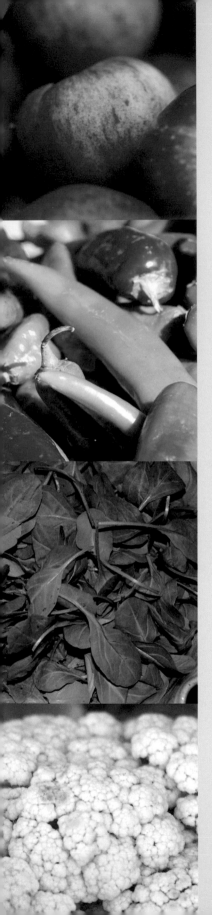

Contents

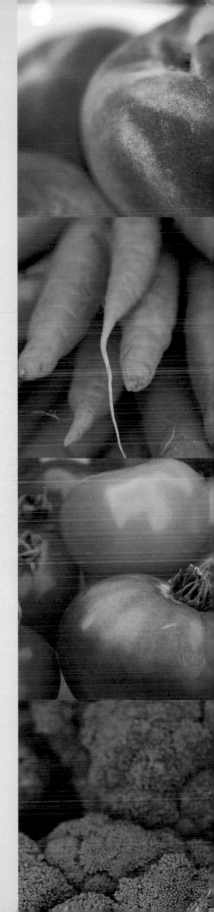

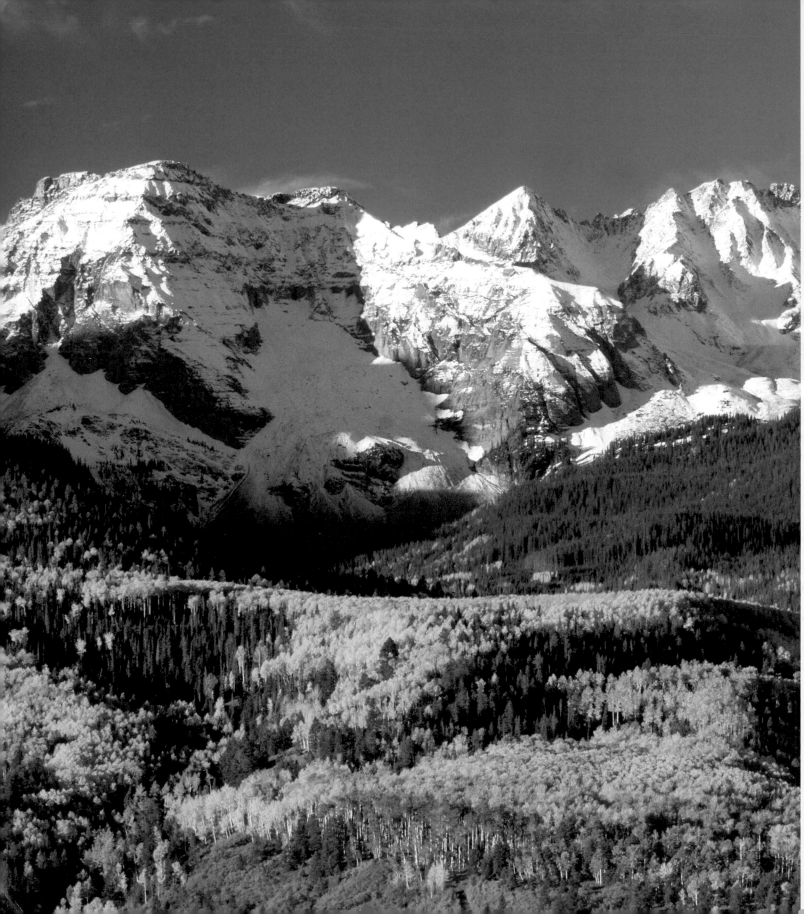

COLORADO FIT KITCHEN
Inspiring Recipes for Mind, Body, Beauty and Optimum Wellness

Dr. James Rouse and Dr. Debra Rouse

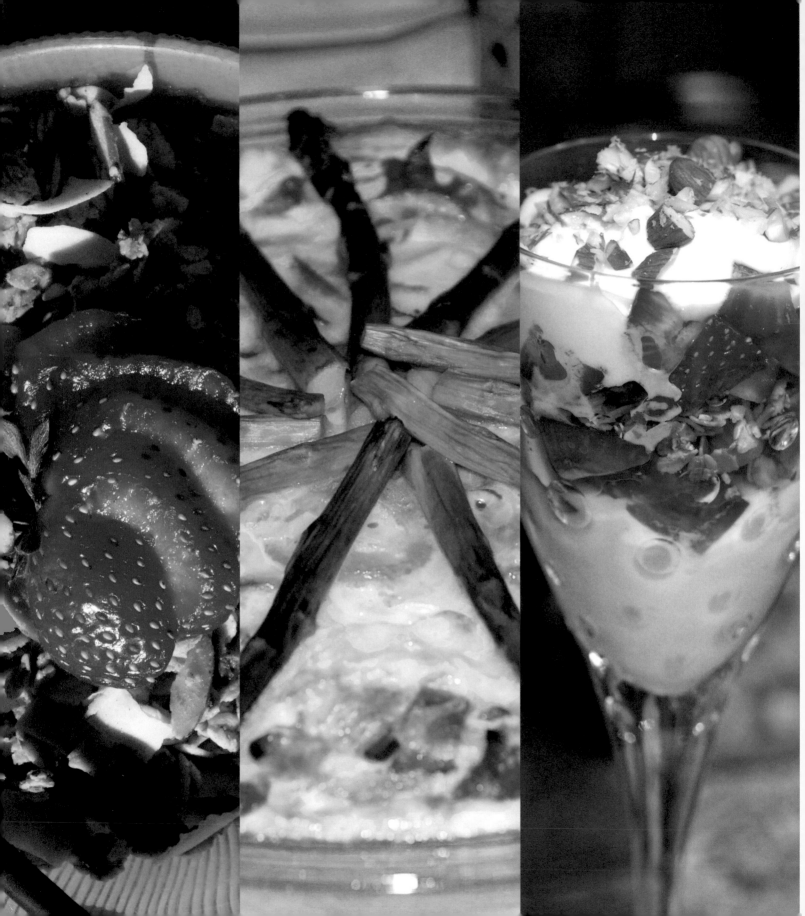

Bountiful Breakfast

Breakfast is definitely an event at our house. What we eat for breakfast sets the tone for the rest of our day. Whether we're feeding kids a healthy breakfast before they head out for school or sports or hosting a brunch – we make sure to begin the day well nourished and balanced from the inside out. Eating breakfast helps kids and adults perform better. The Food Research and Action Center published a nutrition fact sheet that showed that children experiencing hunger have lower math scores and are more likely to repeat a grade. Children and teens who are hungry also display a greater incidence of behavioral, emotional and academic problems.

Breakfast eaters may have an easier time managing their weight. But that doesn't give us license to eat any old thing at breakfast. Remember, food is fuel and if we want to jumpstart the day in a healthy way, we need to eat the right kind of foods in the morning. Beginning the day with high fiber, low glycemic foods, whole grains, healthy fats and adequate protein keeps hunger pangs at bay and actually plays an important role in weight management. People who skip breakfast tend to overeat more throughout the rest of the day.

When we add protein to our morning rituals, we set ourselves up for greater success later in the day. This is especially important for children and young adults. The brain needs fuel first thing in the morning to help all those synapses fire properly. Kids burn a lot of fuel right from the get go, making breakfast so very important.

Not big on breakfast? Start small. Keep hard boiled eggs in the refrigerator so that they are easy to grab and go. Prepare little baggies of whole grain cereal combined with nuts, seeds, and a few pieces of dried fruit like prunes, raisins, or cranberries.

If you tend to skip breakfast, ask yourself why. It only takes a few minutes to prepare heart- and waistline- healthy choices like the ones suggested in our cookbook. Plan ahead, take the time and enjoy all the benefits!

This is an easy dish to prepare for a brunch without the hassle of preparing a crust as we would for a quiche. It is loaded with vitamins, minerals, and protein and also reheats well if you are serving just a few. We'll sometimes make this for dinner when we want something easy and healthy at the same time.

Serves 6

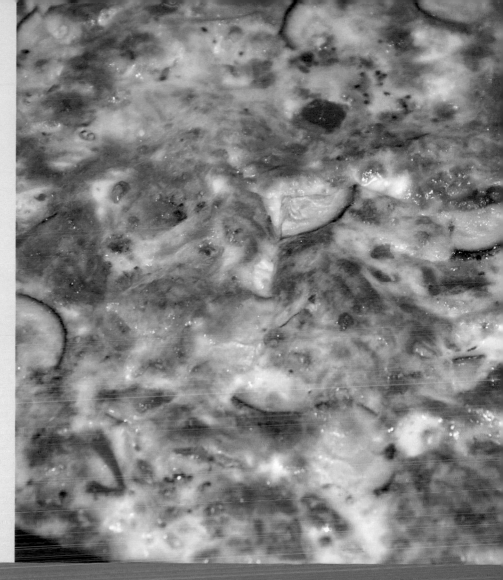

Per Serving:
105 Calories;
8g Fat (3g sat);
10g Protein;
5g Carbohydrate;
1g Dietary Fiber;
216mg Cholesterol;
146mg Sodium.

Boulder Baked Omelet

1 tablespoon olive oil
2 tablespoons onion, finely chopped
1½ cups chopped broccoli
1 cup chopped zucchini
1 medium tomato, coarsely chopped
½ cup lowfat cheddar cheese
½ cup lowfat 2% milk
6 eggs
salt and pepper, as desired
Cooking spray

Preheat oven to 350°F. Meanwhile on the stovetop, sauté onion in olive oil in small cast-iron skillet (or other oven-friendly cooking pan) over medium heat. After about 3 minutes, add broccoli, zucchini and tomatoes and stir-fry another 3 minutes. Layer cheese on top of broccoli, zucchini, and tomatoes. Beat milk, eggs, salt, and pepper until smooth; pour over vegetable mixture.

Bake uncovered until egg mixture is set, 35 to 40 minutes. Let stand 10 minutes before cutting

Breakfast Burritos

Serves 4

8 eggs or 2 cups egg whites or
    egg substitute
½ cup diced green chiles
4 tablespoons shredded lowfat
    mozzarella cheese
½ cup pinto beans, cooked, whole or
    lowfat refried
4 whole wheat tortillas (7- to 8-inch),
    warmed
Options: ½ cup salsa, sliced avocado

Per Serving:
348 Calories;
14g Fat (4g sat);
21g Protein;
35g Carbohydrate;
4g Dietary Fiber;
428mg Cholesterol;
699mg Sodium.

Whisk together eggs or egg substitute in a medium sized bowl.

Prepare a medium (preferably nonstick) skillet over medium heat and coat lightly with cooking spray. Add eggs and cook, stirring frequently until eggs are almost set. Add green chiles and continue to cook until eggs are set.

On another skillet or in the microwave, sprinkle 1 tablespoon of cheese and 2 tablespoon of beans onto the center of each tortilla. Heat until cheese is melted. Remove tortilla to serving plate and top with ¼ of the egg and chile mixture.

Fold the sides of the tortilla over the egg and bean mixture and secure with toothpicks if desired. Serve with salsa and avocado if desired.

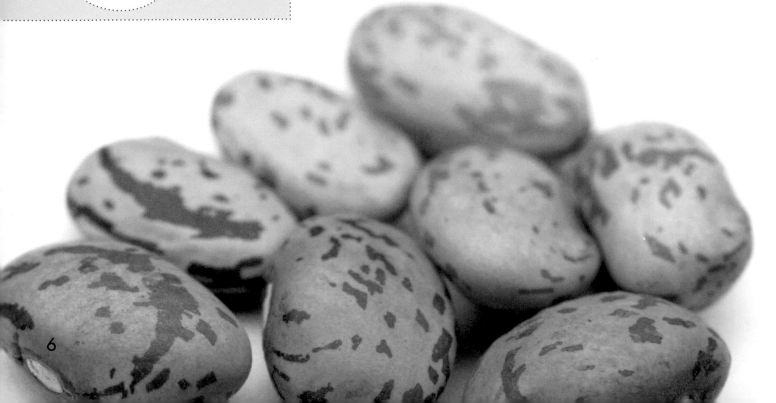

AM-azing cookies

Preheat oven to 350°F (convection bake) or 375°F (normal bake). Combine dry ingredients (oats through ground cinnamon) in a large bowl.

In a medium bowl, combine melted butter with honey, applesauce, milk, and desired extracts.

Combine dry and wet ingredients and mix until just moistened. Drop by heaping tablespoons onto nonstick baking sheet lined with parchment paper. Bake for about 10 minutes or until slightly browned on top.

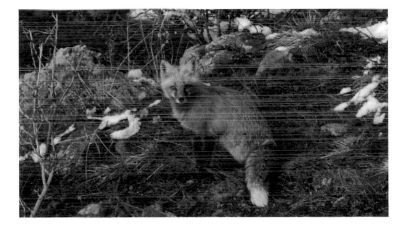

Makes about 24 cookies

2 cups oats
½ cup coconut flour
½ cup amaranth
1 teaspoon baking powder
1 teaspoon baking soda
1 cup walnuts (toasted and chopped)
¼ cup flax seeds, ground
¼ cup dried blueberries
½ teaspoon ground cinnamon
½ cup agave nectar (may substitute honey)
¼ cup melted butter
½ cup applesauce
½ cup lowfat milk, or soy milk
¼ teaspoon maple extract, optional
¼ teaspoon vanilla extract

Per Serving
(2 cookies)
178 Calories; 7g Fat
(2g sat); 5g Protein;
25g Carbohydrate;
5g Dietary Fiber;
5mg Cholesterol;
78mg Sodium.

Did You Know?

Eating oats has been shown to help reduce LDL cholesterol, and lower the risk of developing high blood pressure, obesity, and type 2 diabetes. Beta-glucans from oats and oat fiber may help keep blood sugar levels stable. Oats are a good source of magnesium, selenium, fiber, protein, and vitamin B1 (thiamin). Recent research shows that gluten-sensitive individuals may tolerate oats. Gluten-free rolled oats are available as well.

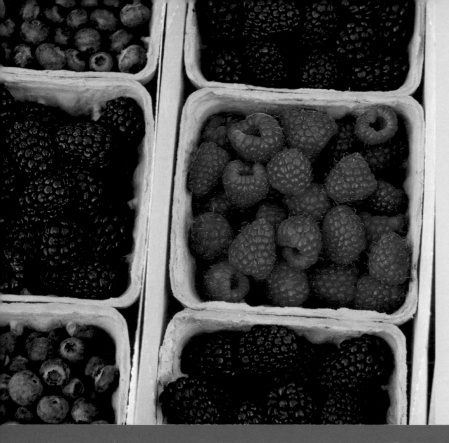

This is a little bit like the morning parfait minus the granola. The lemon-lime combination gives the yogurt a wonderfully tart, yet sweet flavor and the peels contain vitamins and compounds that have been reported to have positive health benefits including cholesterol lowering and insulin resistance-lowering effects. The berries pack a powerful antioxidant and fiber punch and the yogurt with its beneficial probiotics and protein make this an overall outstanding way to begin the day – or eat as a midday snack for lasting energy. We recommend the Greek-style yogurt due to its higher protein content.

Serves 4

Berry Good Breakfast

Whisk together yogurt, honey, juices and peels in a medium size bowl.

Divide fruit between 4 goblets or parfait glasses (approximately ½ cup fruit per serving). Spoon approximately ¼ cup of yogurt sauce over each.

SAUCE
1 cup plain, natural, lowfat or nonfat
  (Greek-style) yogurt
¼ cup honey
2 teaspoons lemon juice, fresh squeezed
2 teaspoons lime juice, fresh squeezed
½ teaspoon lemon peel, finely shredded
½ teaspoon lime peel, finely shredded
½ cup fresh strawberries, sliced
½ cup fresh blueberries
½ cup fresh raspberries
½ cup blackberries

Per Serving:
141 Calories; 1g Fat
(1g sat); 7g Protein;
28g Carbohydrate;
3g Dietary Fiber;
5mg Cholesterol;
28mg Sodium.

8

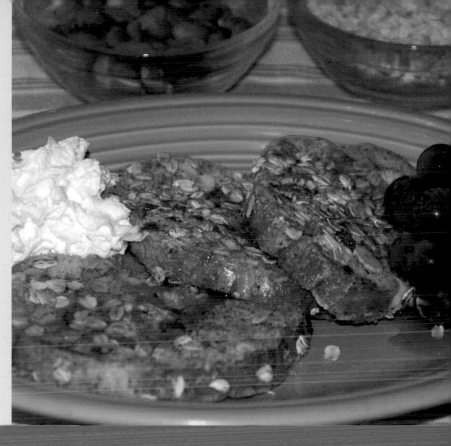

Our kids absolutely love this version of French Toast – they think it tastes like coffee cake! With the added fiber and healthy fats from the nuts, it is a great way to start the day off strong.

Serves 4

Mountain Top Toast

4 large eggs
1 teaspoon vanilla extract
1 cup lowfat milk
½ teaspoon cinnamon
½ teaspoon nutmeg
8 slices French bread (or substitute whole
   grain bread of choice)
½ cup ground almonds
½ cup rolled oats
4 tablespoons maple syrup

Per Serving
(2 slices) :
423 Calories; 18g Fat
(3g sat); 20g Protein;
51g Carbohydrate;
7g Dietary Fiber;
212mg Cholesterol;
376mg Sodium.

Preheat nonstick griddle over medium heat. Crack eggs into a pie plate, add vanilla and whisk until smooth. Whisk in the milk and spices. When well blended, place bread slices into the mixture.

Spread almonds and oats out on another plate. Lay soaked bread in almond-oat mixture and coat well. Turn the bread over and coat the other side.

Spray the griddle with cooking oil spray and carefully place the coated bread down on the prepared griddle. Cook over medium heat for about 4 minutes on each side. Serve hot with real maple syrup.

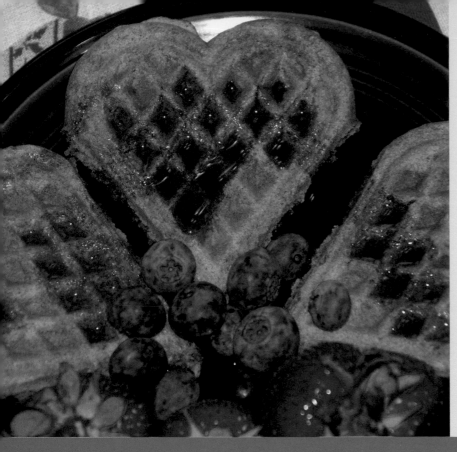

Here's a great recipe for our gluten-free friends. These are substantial and filling waffles with wonderful heart- and waistline-healthy ingredients.

Makes about 6

Per Serving:
163 Calories per waffle. 5g Fat (1g sat - depends on type of milk & yogurt used), 6g Protein; 25 g Carbohydrate, 3g Dietary Fiber; 4mg Cholesterol; 139mg Sodium.

Skinny Waffles

Preheat waffle iron and coat with nonstick cooking spray.

Whisk together dry ingredients (flour through baking soda) in large bowl. In medium bowl, whisk milk, yogurt, oil and eggs. Combine wet and dry ingredients until just mixed. If batter appears too thick, slowly add more milk.

Ladle or spoon about ⅓ cup batter into waffle iron, close lid and cook until golden.

1 cup buckwheat flour
1 cup rice flour
3 tablespoons flax seeds (ground)
1½ teaspoons ground cinnamon
¾ teaspoon baking soda
1 cup soy milk, rice milk, or buttermilk
1 cup yogurt (plain or vanilla)
1 tablespoon vegetable oil
3 eggs

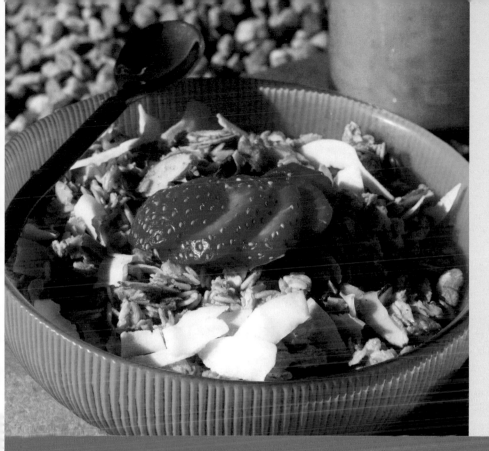

This granola is a guaranteed crowd pleaser. It is a staple in our pantry at home and we often make big batches of it during the holiday season and give it as gifts. If you triple the recipe, you'll make about 4 quart-sized mason jars full and have some extra left over that you and your family can enjoy.

Makes about 8 servings

Per Serving
(½ cup):
426 Calories;
19g Fat (3g sat); 13g Protein;
53g Carbohydrate;
8g Dietary Fiber;
0mg Cholesterol;
12mg Sodium.

Grateful Granola

Preheat oven to 325°F. Mix together oats, wheat germ (or flax), nuts, and cinnamon in large bowl. Add oil, syrup, and extract and stir until well mixed. Divide mixture in half and spread evenly across 1 or 2 ungreased cookie sheets (should have at least a ½ inch "lip" on the side of the cookie sheet to prevent spills; technically called a jelly roll pan). Bake for about 20 minutes or until slightly browned. Allow to cool and stir in dried coconut. Store in airtight containers and enjoy!

3 cups rolled oats (we use the certified gluten-free oats)
½ cup wheat germ or ground flax seed
½ cup slivered almonds
¼ cup sunflower seeds
1 teaspoon ground cinnamon
¼ cup canola oil
¼ cup agave syrup (or sub honey or maple syrup)
½ teaspoon almond extract (can sub maple extract if preferred)
½ teaspoon vanilla extract
¼ cup dried coconut, shredded or flakes

Optional: Dried or fresh fruits (currants, berries, raisins, larger coconut pieces)

There is a lot of flexibility in this recipe. For example, you may substitute buckwheat flour for the chestnut or teff flour. You could use potato flour or starch in place of the tapioca flour. We like to add a scoop of protein powder to give the pancakes an added boost of protein. The vanilla whey protein also makes the pancakes fluffy with a sweet flavor. You can also leave this out and just add a few additional tablespoons of flour or substitute dry milk powder.

Serves 4

½ cup brown rice flour
½ cup gluten-free rolled oats
¼ cup teff flour, coconut flour, or chestnut flour
¼ cup tapioca flour
1 scoop whey vanilla protein powder (optional)
2 tablespoons ground flaxseed
1 teaspoon baking powder
1 dash sea salt
1 dash cinnamon
2 eggs
1 cup lowfat milk
2 tablespoons melted butter or canola oil
½ teaspoon gluten-free vanilla extract (optional)
Cooking oil spray for skillet

Per Serving
(2 pancakes):
326 Calories; 14g Fat
(2g sat); 14g Protein;
47g Carbohydrate;
4g Dietary Fiber;
109mg Cholesterol;
237mg Sodium.

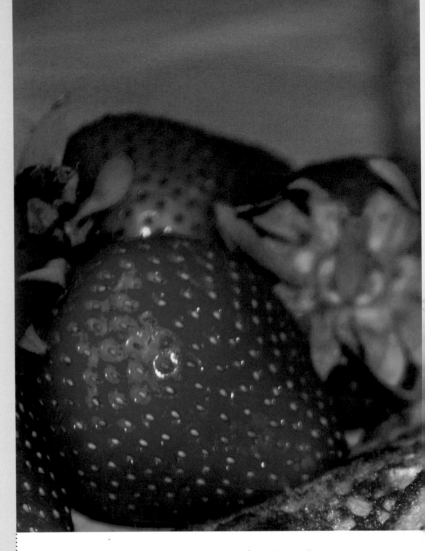

Whisk together dry ingredients (rice flour through cinnamon) in large mixing bowl.

Preheat nonstick skillet to medium-high or lightly coat a large skillet with cooking oil spray.

In a separate bowl or large glass measuring cup, whisk together the wet ingredients (eggs through vanilla). Add wet ingredients to dry and whisk or

Against the Grain Pancakes

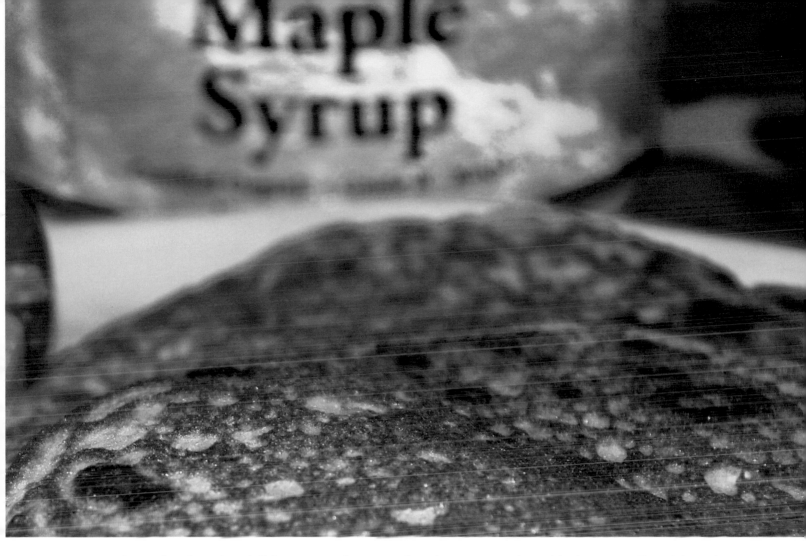

stir together until well combined. If thinner pancakes are preferred you may need to add a bit more milk until desired consistency is reached.

Ladle about ⅓ cup batter for each pancake either into a circle or whatever fun shape you desire. Flip when you begin to see little bubbles appearing in the batter. After flipping, pancakes should be done in about 2 minutes. Serve warm with fresh berries, nut butter and real maple syrup.

For waffles, ladle or spoon about ⅔ cup batter into waffle iron, close lid and cook until golden.

Muy Buenos Huevos

In a small saucepan, combine refried beans with water, minced onions and garlic. Heat over low heat and stir until well combined with a nice consistency that isn't too thick or too thin. When you reach this desired consistency, set aside.

In a larger nonstick skillet, heat tortillas, lightly coating each side with cooking oil spray and turning once on each side (about two minutes). Remove from heat and keep warm (you may choose to skip this step and warm the tortillas in the microwave).

Using the same skillet, lightly spray again with the cooking oil spray. Carefully crack each egg (this may be easier to do 2 at a time) and cook "sunny side up" style or if you prefer them scrambled you may do that as well. When the eggs are almost done, you may turn off the heat and assemble the tortillas.

Place 2 tortillas on each plate. Mound about 2 tablespoons of the bean mixture on each tortilla. Place an egg on top of each tortilla and top with about 2 tablespoons of the green chili sauce and sprinkle with avocado and about a tablespoon of shredded cheese as desired.

Here is an outstanding brunch or "breakfast for dinner" recipe. We love the terrific flavors and awesome nutritionals with fiber and antioxidants in the beans and tortillas, vitamin C in the chiles, and health-promoting sulfur compounds in the onions and garlic. Olé!

Serves 4

1 cup lowfat refried beans
1 tablespoon water
½ cup medium red onion, minced
2 garlic cloves, minced
8 whole grain flour tortillas (such as "Fat Flush") or Sprouted Corn Tortillas
8 eggs, (or egg whites) nonstick cooking oil spray
½ cup green chile sauce/salsa (we love 505 Southwestern)
optional: ½ avocado, diced, ½ cup shredded nonfat mozzarella cheese

Per Serving
(using "Fat Flush tortillas," whole eggs, cheese and avocados):
520 Calories; 17g Fat (3g sat); 37g Protein; 54g Carbohydrate; 16g Dietary Fiber; 429mg Cholesterol; 878mg Sodium.

(without avocado or cheese) Per Serving:
479 Calories; 17g Fat; 28g Protein; 53g Carbohydrate; 16g Dietary Fiber; 424mg Cholesterol; 656mg Sodium.

(using egg whites and without avocado or cheese) Per Serving:
365 Calories; 7g Fat; 23g Protein; 53g Carbohydrate; 16g Dietary Fiber; 0mg Cholesterol; 625mg Sodium.

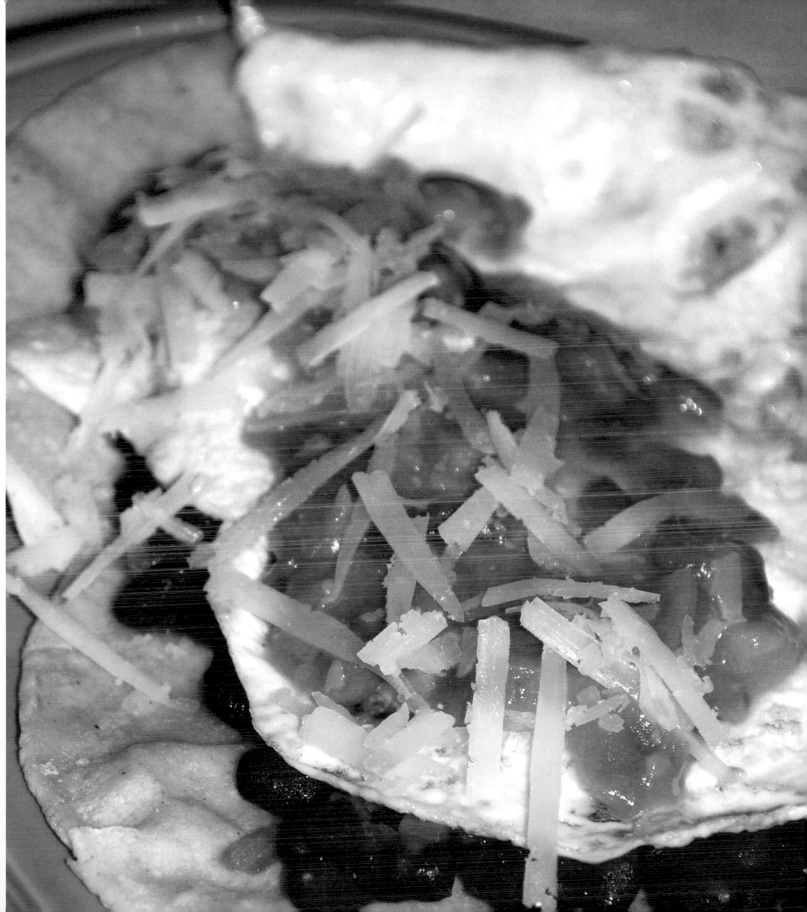

Preheat waffle iron and spray lightly with cooking spray. Whisk together dry ingredients (flour through salt) in large bowl. In medium bowl, whisk milk, peppers, cilantro, oil and eggs. Combine wet and dry ingredients and stir together until just mixed.

Ladle or spoon about ⅓ cup batter into waffle iron, close lid and cook until golden brown.

Per Serving:
149 Calories
per waffle. 4g Fat,
(1g sat), 4g Protein;
17g Carbohydrate,
1g Dietary Fiber,
3mg Cholesterol,
542mg Sodium

You can also make these into pancakes and serve along side a Southwestern-themed dinner. They go great with Huevos Rancheros!

Makes about 6 depending on the size of your waffle iron

1 cup unbleached flour
¾ cup cornmeal
1 teaspoon ground cumin
¾ teaspoon baking soda
1½ teaspoons salt
1½ cups soymilk or buttermilk
2 medium jalapeno peppers, minced and seeded (you
    may want to wear gloves for this preparation)
2 tablespoons minced fresh cilantro
1 tablespoon vegetable oil
2 eggs

Wicked Hot Waffles

Jalapeno chile peppers not only contain a lot of vitamin C, but they contain a powerful chemical called capsaicin, which is responsible for all the heat. Capsaicin may provide pain relief for headaches, help combat sinusitis and congestion, act as a natural anti-inflammatory agent, and help rev up our metabolic engines. Topical capsaicin may be used to ease the pain of arthritis and shingles (must not be used over any open lesions or ouch!!).

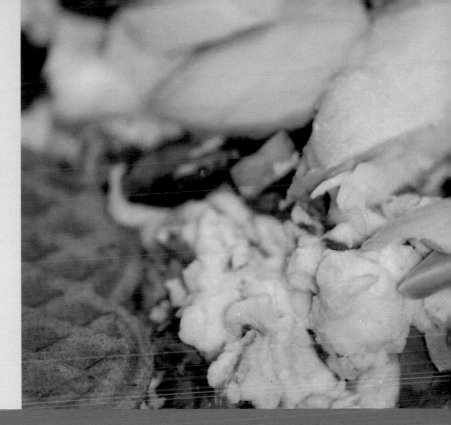

Truth be told, James has this for breakfast most days. During the winter he may substitute steel cut oats for the waffle and on weekends he'll dive into a frittata, Huevos Rancheros, or some kind of wonderful baked goody. He tends to add tons of vegetables so feel free to expand your pulate here beyond the baby spinach. Adding veggies to your eggs first thing in the morning is a great strategy for reaching your goal of getting five to nine servings of fruits and vegetables daily (and if this hasn't been one of your goals, it's time to make it one!). Add ½ grapefruit to this breakfast and you'll be that much closer to reaching your goal!

James' Eggceptional Breakfast

Serves 1

2 eggs
2 egg whites
½ teaspoon olive oil
½ cup chopped fresh baby spinach leaves
Sea salt and pepper, to taste
1 Skinny Waffle (p. 10)
1 teaspoon almond butter

Optional: ¼ avocado sliced

Per Serving:
348 Calories;
19g Fat (4g sat);
21g Protein;
22g Carbohydrate;
1g Dietary Fiber;
424mg Cholesterol;
477mg Sodium.

Whisk egg and egg whites together. Heat a skillet over medium heat and add ½ teaspoon of olive oil. Add egg mixture and stir with spatula until eggs are nearly cooked through. Add spinach and continue stirring and cooking eggs until spinach is well incorporated and eggs are fully cooked. Season with salt and pepper as desired and top with sliced avocado.

James usually has this with a Skinny Waffle topped with almond butter.

Granola Splits

Pretty to look at, luscious to eat!

Serves 4

2 cups lowfat yogurt (again we recommend plain Greek-style)
2 cups chopped strawberries
½ cup granola
4 tablespoons chopped almonds

Alternate layers of fruit, granola, and ¼ cup yogurt in 4 goblets or parfait glasses, beginning and ending with either fruit or yogurt. Top with 1 tablespoon chopped almonds.

Per Serving:
195 Calories;
9g Fat (1g sat);
15g Protein;
16g Carbohydrate;
3g Dietary Fiber;
10mg Cholesterol;
55mg Sodium.

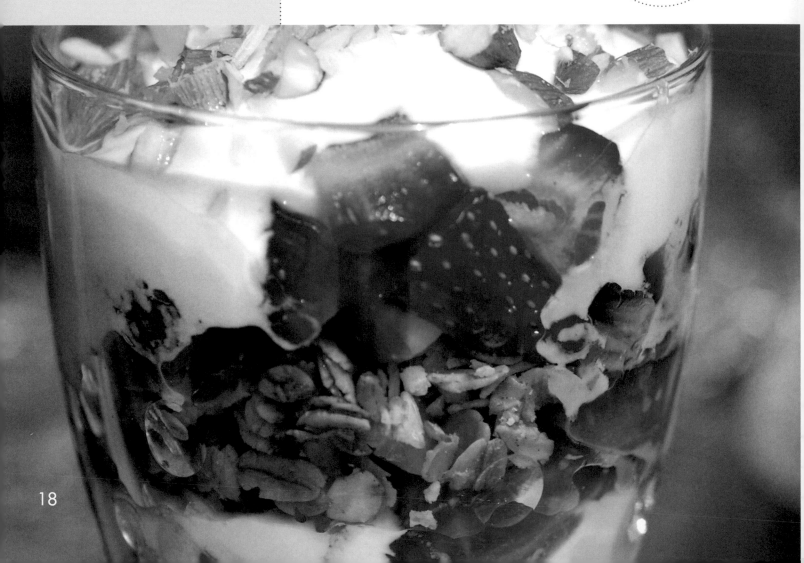

18

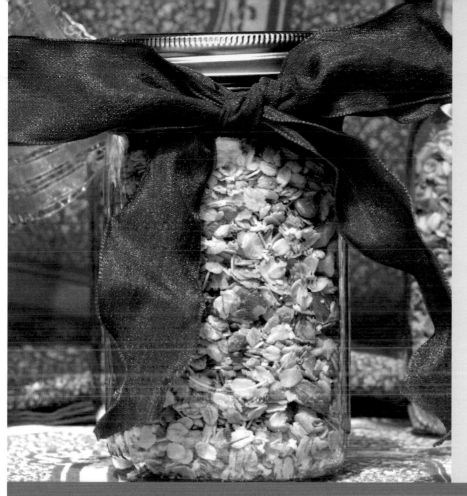

If you love nuts like we do, then you'll love this version of granola. The Vermonter in James appreciates the incredible maple flavor in this version as well. Experiment with adding dried fruit like organic dried blueberries or currants, after you've baked the granola.

Serves 14

Per Serving
(14 cup)
288 Calories; 16g Fat
(1g sat); 8g Protein;
31g Carbohydrate;
5g Dietary Fiber;
0 mg Cholesterol;
3 mg Sodium.

Groovy Granola

Preheat oven to 325°F. Mix together oats, nuts, and cinnamon in large bowl. Add oil, syrup, maple flavor and stir until well mixed. Divide mixture in half and spread evenly across 2 ungreased cookie sheets (should have at least a ½ inch "lip" on the side of the cookie sheet to prevent spills). Bake for about 20 minutes or until slightly browned. Allow to cool and then add dried fruit and mix again. Store in airtight containers and enjoy!

6 cups organic rolled oats
½ cup (each) chopped almonds, hazelnuts, walnuts
⅓ cup organic canola oil
⅓ cup organic maple syrup
½ teaspoon maple flavor (frontier spices)
1 teaspoon cinnamon

Optional: ½ cup wheat germ or ¼ cup ground flax seed
Other Options: dried blueberries, cranberries, apples

Fully Committed Cinnamon Rolls

A Christmas morning tradition in the Rouse house. Everyone deserves a little indulgence and we've made these cinnamon rolls about as healthy as they come.

Makes 15

3½ cups whole wheat flour, divided
⅓ cup granulated sugar
1 teaspoon salt
1 package active dry yeast (2¼ tsp)
1 cup lowfat 1% milk, warm
⅓ cup melted ghee (or butter)
  or regular butter
1 egg, slightly beaten

Filling
2 tablespoons softened butter or ghee
3 tablespoons packed brown sugar
1 teaspoon ground cinnamon
¾ cup apples, chopped
¾ cup walnuts, chopped
1 whisked egg, for wash

Per Serving:
323 Calories;
21g Fat (11g sat);
7g Protein;
31g Carbohydrate;
4g Dietary Fiber;
57mg Cholesterol;
162mg Sodium.

Whisk together 2 cups of the flour, ⅓ cup granulated sugar, salt and yeast in a large bowl. Add warm milk, ⅓ cup ghee (or butter) and slightly beaten egg.

Beat on low speed 1 minute, scraping bowl frequently. Stir in enough remaining flour, ½ cup at a time, to make dough easy to handle. This is easiest with a stand up mixer and a dough hook.

Turn dough onto lightly floured surface; knead about 5 minutes or until smooth and elastic. Place in a greased bowl; turn greased side up. Cover and let rise in warm place about 1½ hours or until double. Dough is ready if indentation remains when touched.

Lightly coat a rectangular baking dish, 13 × 9 × 2 inches with cooking spray.

Punch down dough. Flatten with hands or use a rolling pin and roll into a rectangle, approximately 15 × 10 inches; spread with 2 tablespoons ghee. Mix together the brown sugar, cinnamon, apples, and walnuts. Sprinkle evenly over rectangle. Roll up tightly, beginning at 15-inch side. Pinch edge of dough into roll to seal. Stretch and shape to make even.

Cut roll into fifteen 1-inch slices. Place slightly apart in pan. Wrap pan with heavy-duty aluminum foil. Refrigerate at least 2 hours but no longer than 48 hours. (To bake immediately, do not wrap. Let rise in warm place about 30 minutes or until double. Then bake as directed.)

Heat oven to 350°F. Brush the top of the rolls with whisked egg. Bake uncovered 30 to 35 minutes or until golden brown.

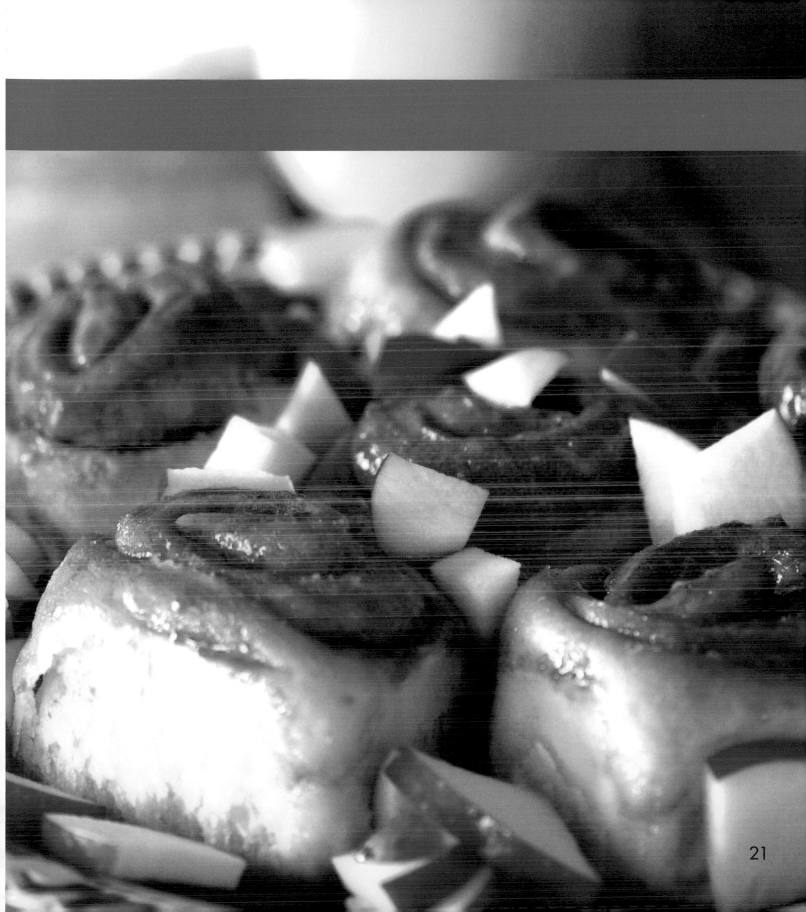

21

Morning Om

Basic but efficient, quick and healthy start to a great day.

Serves 1

2 medium eggs
2 slices whole wheat bread
½ cup chopped spinach
1 teaspoon chives
½ teaspoon butter
salt and pepper as desired

Per Serving:
306 Calories;
14g Fat (5g sat);
18g Protein;
27g Carbohydrate;
4g Dietary Fiber;
429mg Cholesterol;
467mg Sodium.

We always use a nonstick 3-cup egg poacher when we poach eggs. We start with a small amount of water in the bottom of a medium size saucepan. We spray the poaching cups with cooking oil spray and crack the eggs carefully into 2 of the three spots for the eggs. In the third spot, we put the chopped up spinach so it will steam as the eggs do.

Heat the poaching water to boiling (being sure that you do not boil off all of the water or you may scorch the bottom of the pan). Cover the eggs (and spinach) while they are cooking and poach for about 5 to 7 minutes until desired doneness. You can use a fork to pierce the egg a few times while it is cooking to check its progress.

While the eggs are cooking, make your toast and have it ready for serving time. When the eggs are done carefully remove from the poaching pan and slide them along with the spinach onto the toast. Sprinkle chives on top and season with salt and pepper if desired.

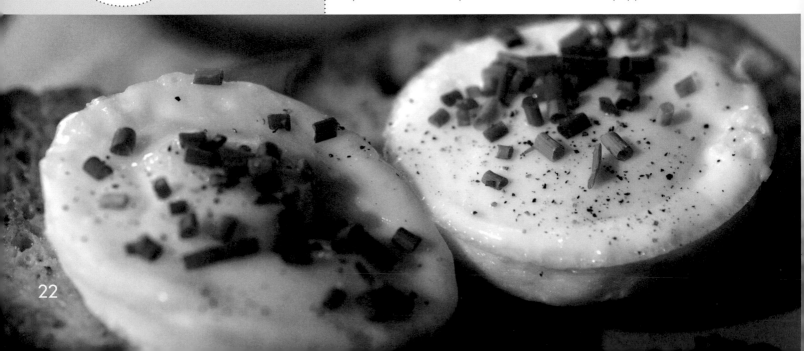

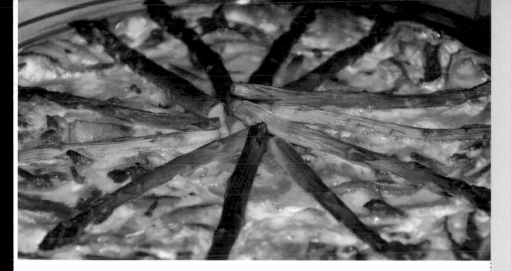

Preheat oven to 350°F. Rinse potatoes well and slice thinly (no bigger than ¼ inch slices). Steam potato slices for about 5 minutes using a steam basket in a large skillet or stock pot. Allow to cool.

In a cast iron skillet or frying pan, sauté red pepper and onion in olive oil until onions are lightly browned. Stir frequently. Using a microwave safe dish, microwave bacon between 2 layers of paper towels for about 3 minutes. When cool enough to handle, chop into thin slices and add to pepper and onion mixture. Sauté this mixture an additional minute or two.

In a medium bowl, whisk together milk, cream, eggs, and egg whites. Whisk in cheese. Season with black pepper.

Layer steamed potatoes in a glass baking dish (pie shaped) coated with cooking spray. Place red pepper, onion and bacon mixture on top of this. Pour milk and egg mixture on top of all of this. Top with asparagus spears.

Bake for 35 minutes. Allow to set and cool at least 10 minutes prior to serving.

Per Serving:
160 Calories;
7g Fat (2g sat);
10g Protein;
14g Carbohydrate;
2g Dietary Fiber;
118mg Cholesterol,
220mg Sodium.

Potatoes are a great alternative to the traditional flour and butter laden crusts. We've lightened up the traditional quiche recipe by adding antioxidant rich vegetables like red bell pepper and asparagus and cutting the fat by using egg whites and turkey bacon. You can also substitute tempeh "fakin bacon" here as we have many times. Look for nitrite-free, natural bacon whenever possible.

Serves 8

1 large russet potato, thinly sliced
1 tablespoon olive oil
½ medium red bell pepper, diced
1 medium onion, thinly sliced
5 pieces turkey bacon slices
½ cup lowfat 1% milk
1 tablespoon heavy cream
4 medium eggs
2 medium egg whites
½ cup lowfat cheddar cheese, grated
1 dash black pepper
12 asparagus spears, lightly steamed

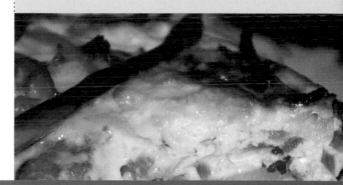

Spud Bob Quiche Pants

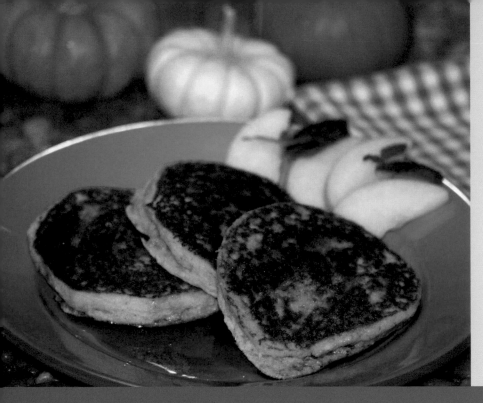

Another favorite fall recipe, our household loves pumpkin pancakes. You can make these as written as a gluten-free pancake, or feel free to substitute with whole wheat or all-purpose flour. We've been known to serve these with dinner in lieu of a "bread basket." They can also be served as dessert with fresh fruit and a dollup of whipped cream.

Serves 4

Fall in Love Pancakes

Whisk flours, sugar, baking powder, spice, and salt in a large bowl until well blended.

In a separate bowl, whisk together milk, eggs, butter, pumpkin purée, and vanilla extract.

Stir or blend dry ingredients into wet. Batter should be a little bit thick. If too thick then stir in more milk, one tablespoon at a time.

Brush a large nonstick skillet with oil or spray with cooking oil spray. Heat to medium high. Pour ⅓ cup of batter onto skillet to form pancake rounds, one at a time. Cook about 2 minutes each side – flipping when bubbles appear on the surface or bottoms of pancakes are brown.

Serve warm with real maple syrup.

1 cup brown rice flour
½ cup coconut flour
1 tablespoon sugar
2 teaspoons baking powder
1 teaspoon pumpkin pie spice
½ teaspoon salt
1¼ cups lowfat 1% milk
2 eggs
2 tablespoons melted butter
½ cup pumpkin purée
1 teaspoon vanilla extract

4 tablespoons maple syrup

Per Serving:
470 Calories;
13g Fat (7g sat);
13g Protein;
75g Carbohydrate;
15g Dietary Fiber;
125mg Cholesterol;
649mg Sodium.

24

Oats are already known for helping remove cholesterol from the digestive system – but did you know oats also contain antioxidants that may strengthen our immune systems and may help reduce our risk for heart failure, high blood pressure and other signs of cardiovascular disease? Beta-glucan in oats may also help stabilize blood sugar levels, thus being beneficial in the prevention and treatment of type 2 diabetes. Steel cut oats are more dense and chewy than rolled oats – and as a result, take a bit longer to cook. Trust us, they're worth the wait.

Serves 4

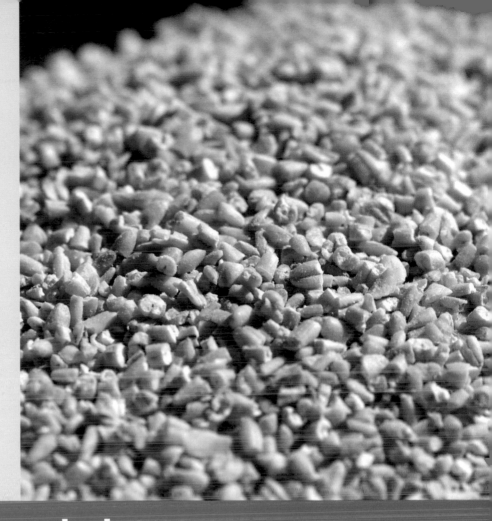

Loaded Oats

1 cup steel cut oats
4 cups water
1 cup apples, chopped
1 teaspoon cinnamon
1 tablespoon brown sugar
1 cup cottage cheese

Per Serving:
299 Calories;
4g Fat (0g sat);
14g Protein;
47g Carbohydrate;
7g Dietary Fiber;
5mg Cholesterol;
238mg Sodium.

Bring water to a boil, stir in steel cut oats, return to a boil and then reduce heat to simmer. Simmer for about 15 minutes. Stir in chopped apples, cinnamon, and brown sugar. Cover and turn off heat. Allow to sit for another 10 minutes covered. Serve warm with a small side of cottage cheese.

Where the Wild Things Are

Serves 8

1½ cups whole wheat flour, or ¾ cup whole
    wheat and ¾ cup all purpose flour
¼ tablespoon salt
4 tablespoons canola oil
3 tablespoons unsalted butter, chilled
4 tablespoons ice water
1 tablespoon olive oil
½ tablespoon unsalted butter
1 cup cremini mushrooms, sliced
1 cup shiitake mushrooms, sliced
1 cup portobello mushrooms, sliced
1 cup shallots, thinly sliced
2 cups arugula leaves
¼ cup gouda cheese
5 eggs
⅔ cup lowfat milk
1 tablespoon heavy cream
1 dash nutmeg
1 dash pepper
½ teaspoon dried thyme

Per Serving:
323 Calories;
21g Fat (11g sat);
7g Protein;
31g Carbohydrate;
4g Dietary Fiber;
57mg Cholesterol;
162mg Sodium.

Combine flour and salt in food processor and pulse several times. Place oil and chilled butter, cut into pieces, into food processor and pulse until a crumb-like substance appears. Add water and pulse until a ball begins to form. (More water may be necessary). Form into a flattened round, cover with plastic wrap and refrigerate for about thirty minutes to an hour.

Preheat oven to 350°F. Roll out dough on a well floured surface, place in an oven-safe pie baking dish. You can also skip the rolling and just press the dough into the pie pan. Prebake the pie crust for about 10 minutes. Remove and set aside until other ingredients are ready.

Use a large skillet to sauté olive oil, shallots and mushrooms over medium high heat. Continue to stir until mushrooms become lightly browned and you notice they have become moist. When nearly done, add arugula leaves and stir-fry for about a minute – until the arugula is wilted.

Place shredded cheese on the bottom of the crust. Top with the mushroom and arugula mixture.

Whisk together eggs, milk, cream and spices. Pour over crust, cheese and veggie mixture. Bake for about 40 minutes until no evidence of liquid remains. Allow to sit about 5 minutes before serving.

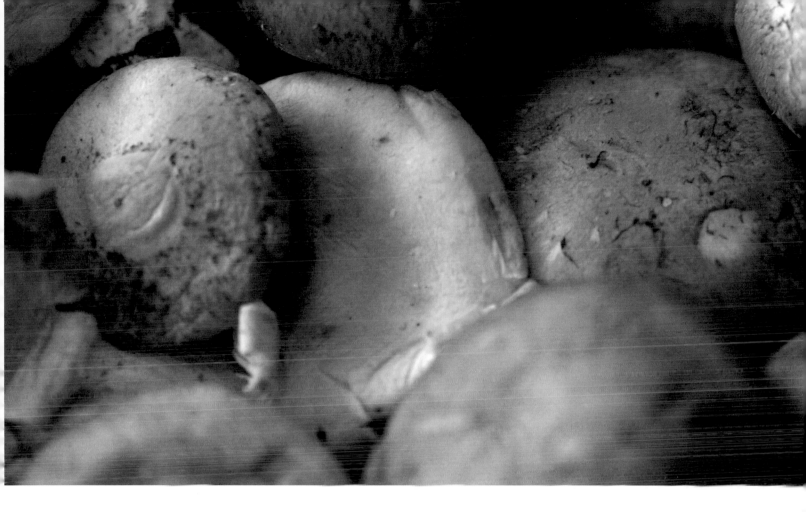

The more indulgent and typical crust is made healthier with the addition of whole wheat flour and canola oil rather than all white flour and butter. This combination of mushrooms lends a wonderfully earthy flavor to the quiche and they bring quality nutrition as well. Cremini mushrooms are a great source of selenium, zinc, and B vitamins. Shiitake mushrooms contain a chemical called lentinan that has a positive effect on the immune system, shown to fight against infections and viruses.

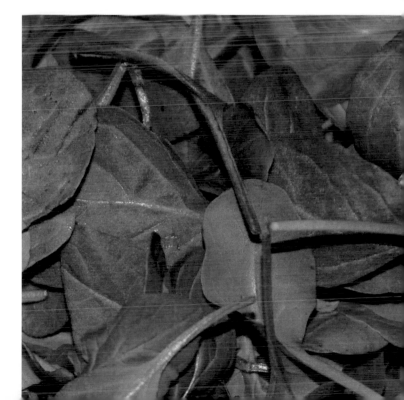

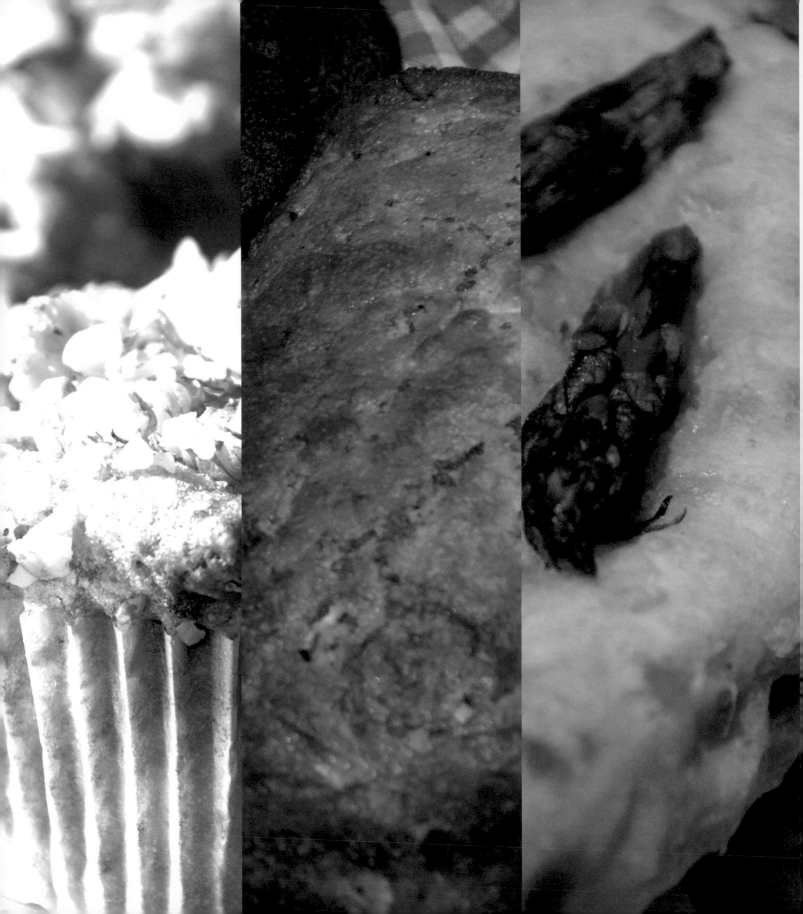

Vegetables are a must on a diet. I suggest carrot cake,
zucchini bread, and pumpkin pie. ~Jim Davis

Baked Goodies

Notes on muffins:

Your muffin tin should always be placed on the center oven rack, in the middle of the rack. Some people like to rotate the muffin tin 90 degrees half way through cooking to allow for more even baking. We seldom do this. The muffins closest to the side of the oven wall tend to cook more quickly compared to those in the center. Personally, Debra goes crazy when anyone opens the oven door while things are baking.

Cooking times and temperatures often vary in different climates, so keep in mind that you may need to adjust depending on where you live. For example, if the recipe calls to bake for 25 minutes, that could mean 20 to 30 minutes for you. We've tried to indicate this in most recipes. Also, where we live at altitude (over 7200 feet), we sometimes have to adjust the recipes a bit, adding a little more liquid or increasing the temperature of our oven. Again, we have attempted to make the recipes as user-friendly as possible.

Also, we like to use environmentally friendly "If You Care" brand natural unbleached baking cups. They don't need any additional greasing of the pan and the muffins don't stick to the paper because it is coated with silicone, a non-organic natural product. To find their products go to www.ifyoucare.com.

Most of these recipes can be made gluten-free and/or vegan. All we do is substitute any wheat or all-purpose flour with ¾ brown rice flour and ¼ coconut flour (or a combination of coconut and tapioca flour). Vegans can feel free to use egg replacer powder (www.ener-g.com) and dairy-free buttery spreads from companies like Earth Balance (www.earthbalancenatural.com).

We made these muffins daily for the Common Sense Café in Portland, Oregon. You can double the recipe for larger muffins with big muffin tops – and during the fall apple harvest, use your homemade applesauce and these will be extra delicious.

Makes 12

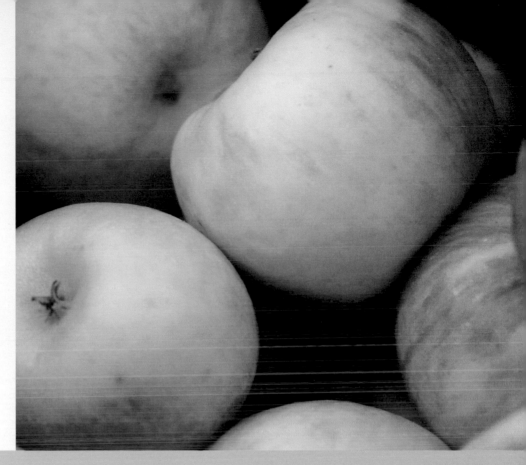

Common Sense Café Muffins

¼ cup canola oil
¼ cup maple syrup
1 cup applesauce
1½ cups whole wheat pastry flour
½ teaspoon baking soda
1 teaspoon baking powder
¾ teaspoon cinnamon
1 pinch sea salt
½ cup chopped walnuts

Per Muffin:
161 Calories;
8g Fat (1g sat);
3g Protein;
21g Carbohydrate;
3g Dietary Fiber;
0mg Cholesterol;
104mg Sodium.

Preheat oven to 375°F. Lightly coat a 12-cup muffin tin with cooking spray or paper liners.

Combine oil, maple syrup, and applesauce in a medium size bowl. Stir to mix. In a separate bowl, sift together the flour, baking soda and powders, cinnamon, and salt. Stir in walnuts. Combine wet and dry ingredients and stir until just combined. Use a large spoon to drop the muffin batter into the muffin tins. Bake for 18 to 20 minutes.

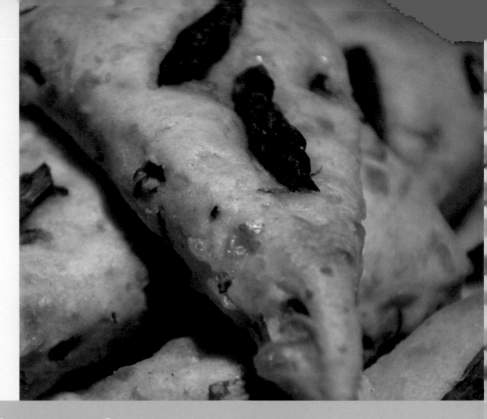

These savory scones have an unexpected lingering spice that is sure to surprise and please the palate. They pair great with soups and salads. Enjoy when asparagus is at its peak – mid Spring through Summer.

Makes 8-10

Enlightened Scones

½ pound steamed asparagus
1 cup all purpose flour
1 cup whole wheat pastry flour
1 tablespoon baking powder
½ teaspoon salt
4 tablespoons unsalted butter
¾ cup plus 2 tablespoons lowfat milk or
   buttermilk
1 cup grated lowfat cheddar cheese
½ teaspoon cayenne pepper
¼ teaspoon black pepper

Per Serving:
203 Calories;
8g Fat (4g sat);
8g Protein;
26g Carbohydrate;
3g Dietary Fiber;
20mg Cholesterol;
415mg Sodium.

Preheat oven to 425°F. Trim tips from asparagus, and chop stalks into ¼-inch pieces. *Stir together flour, baking powder and salt in large bowl. Cut butter into small pieces. Using fingers, rub butter into flour mixture until mixture resembles coarse meal. Stir in ¾ cup milk. Fold in cheese, asparagus pieces (but not tips), cayenne and pepper. Dough might be sticky.

Turn dough onto floured work surface, and knead 6 or 7 times. Incorporate enough flour to make smooth and easy to shape. Shape dough into one large round or 2 smaller rounds. Using sharp knife, cut into triangles (ideally 8 to12 scones total). Place triangles on greased or parchment lined baking sheet. Brush scones with remaining tablespoon of buttermilk, them press 2 or 3 asparagus tips into tops. Bake 12 to 15 minutes, or until tops are golden brown.

*This can be done in a stand-up mixer.

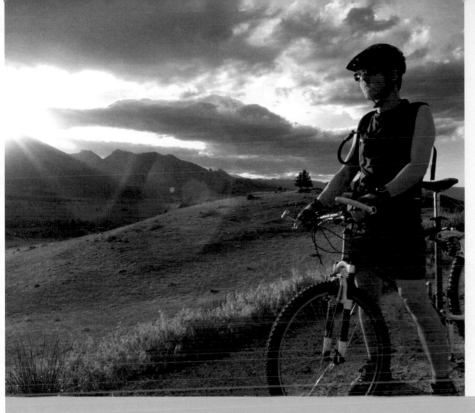

These muffins are wonderfully filling and naturally sweet. We like to have them with an egg or two to up the protein first thing in the morning. Or enjoy them with a glass of your favorite kind of milk and you'll be off to a healthy start.

Makes 12

Hit the Trail Muffins

Preheat oven to 350°F. Line muffin pan with muffin liners or lightly coat with cooking spray.

Beat the banana, sugar, oil, and eggs until well combined.

Whisk together flour, flaxseed meal, baking powder, baking soda and salt. Gradually add dry mixture to banana mixture and stir together until ingredients are just mixed. Stir in chopped dates. Fill muffin tins ½ to ¾ full with batter.

Bake for 25 minutes or until a toothpick inserted in the center comes out clean. Remove to a wire rack and let the muffins cool slightly before removing them from muffin cup.

1½ banana, mashed
½ cup sugar
¼ cup canola oil
2 eggs
1½ cups whole wheat pastry flour
½ cup flax seed, ground into meal
½ teaspoon baking powder
½ teaspoon baking soda
¼ teaspoon sea salt
½ cup dates, pitted and chopped

Per Serving:
222 Calories; 8g Fat
(1g sat); 4g Protein;
35g Carbohydrate;
4g Dietary Fiber;
35mg Cholesterol;
128mg Sodium.

33

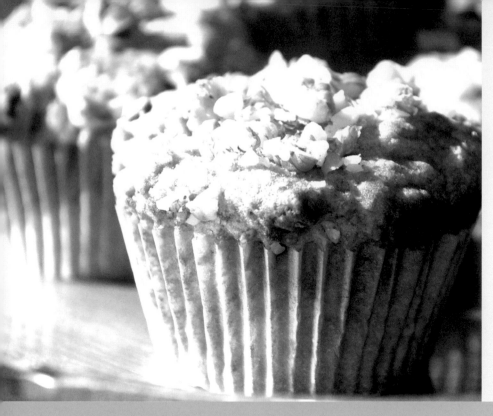

These muffins are probably the kids' favorites. Adding a scoop of protein powder is a fun little strategy we use to sneak a little more protein into the diet. You can always leave out the protein powder and replace it with the same amount of flour or dry milk powder if desired. The chocolate chips blend well with all of the other flavors and these muffins are sure to satisfy folks of all ages.

Makes 12

Funky Monkey Muffins

Preheat oven to 400°F. In a food processor fitted with steel blade, add ¼ cup walnuts and pulse until crumbly. Add flour, oat bran, baking powder, baking soda, cinnamon, and protein powder and continue to pulse until well mixed.

In a large bowl, using an electric mixer, beat together honey, eggs, oil, vanilla extract, mashed bananas, yogurt and milk. Gently fold dry ingredients into the wet. Stir in ¼ cup mini chocolate chips. Do not over mix.

Divide mixture into 12 non-stick muffin pans (or muffin tins lined with paper muffin cups). Sprinkle about 2 teaspoons of chopped walnuts on top of each muffin.

Bake at 400°F for about 5 minutes, reduce heat to 350F for an additional 10 to 15 minutes, until a toothpick comes out clean when inserted in the center.

½ cup chopped walnuts, divided
1½ cups whole wheat pastry flour
½ cup oat bran
½ teaspoon baking powder
½ teaspoon baking soda
1 teaspoon ground cinnamon
2 tablespoons protein powder
¼ cup honey
2 small eggs
¼ cup canola oil
1 teaspoon vanilla extract
2 medium bananas, mashed
¼ cup lowfat yogurt
¼ cup lowfat 1% milk
¼ cup mini-chocolate chips

Per Serving:
222 Calories;
10g Fat (2g sat);
7g Protein;
29g Carbohydrate;
3g Dietary Fiber;
37mg Cholesterol;
99mg Sodium.

34

Memory Muffins

It is easy to grind your own flaxseeds in a common coffee grinder, although it is almost as easy to find it pre-ground for our convenience. We still prefer to grind it ourselves, ensuring that the resulting flaxseed meal is at its freshest. These are very flavorful muffins with loads of healthy ingredients that you can feel good about eating. Great for an afternoon tea or brunch buffet! If you use melted butter, the muffins will be a bit cakier, versus using the oil, which makes it more bread-like. Feel free to substitute applesauce for a lowfat version.

Makes 12

¼ cup ground flaxseed
1 cup whole wheat pastry flour
1 cup all-purpose flour
1 scoop whey protein powder
1 teaspoon baking powder
1 teaspoon ground cinnamon
½ teaspoon salt
1 egg
½ cup maple syrup
2 tablespoons orange juice
¼ cup canola oil or melted butter
½ cup lowfat milk of choice
1½ cups fresh blueberries
½ cup walnuts (optional)
1 tablespoon cinnamon sugar (optional)

We find that the type of milk people drink and prefer varies considerably. In general, for most of our recipes feel free to substitute your milk of choice be it nonfat, lowfat, whole, cow's, goat's, soy, hemp, almond—you get the picture. We highly recommend that whatever milk you do choose, go organic to avoid any unnecessary exposure to pesticides, hormones, or genetically modified organisms.

Preheat oven to 350°F. Lightly coat twelve 2-½-inch muffin cups with cooking oil spray or line with baking cups.

In a large bowl whisk together ground flaxseed, flours, protein powder, baking powder, cinnamon, and salt; set aside.

In a medium bowl beat or whisk the egg. Whisk in the maple syrup, orange juice, oil (or melted butter) and milk. Stir into flour mixture until just combined (batter will be lumpy). Gently fold in blueberries and nuts until evenly distributed. Fill muffin cups ⅔ full with batter. Sprinkle with cinnamon sugar if desired. Bake until top springs back and golden, about 20 minutes.

Per Serving:
228 Calories;
10g Fat (1g sat);
7g Protein;
30g Carbohydrate;
4g Dietary Fiber;
29mg Cholesterol;
185mg Sodium.

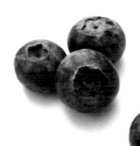

We used to call these carrot cake muffins, but decided to take the cake part out since these muffins can be enjoyed anytime, anywhere. Sure, for decadent times we've been known to add a little layer of frosting. Sometimes we'll have a carrot muffin with a bowl of Greek-style yogurt and call it breakfast!

Makes 18

1 ¼ cups all-purpose flour
1 cup whole wheat pastry flour
1 teaspoon baking powder
¼ teaspoon baking soda
1 teaspoon ground cinnamon
¼ teaspoon ground nutmeg
½ cup sugar
½ cup brown sugar
½ cup applesauce
½ cup dried coconut, shredded
⅓ cup canola oil
¼ cup nonfat vanilla yogurt
1 tablespoon vanilla extract
2 large egg whites
1 large egg
2 cups shredded carrots

Per Serving:
164 Calories;
5g Fat (29.9% calories from fat); 3g Protein;
26g Carbohydrate;
2g Dietary Fiber;
12mg Cholesterol;
70mg Sodium.

Preheat oven to 375°F. Line 18 muffin tins with paper muffin cup liners.

Whisk together flours, baking powder, baking soda, cinnamon and nutmeg in a medium size bowl.

In a separate bowl, beat together sugars, applesauce, dried coconut, canola oil, yogurt, vanilla extract, egg whites and eggs. Stir the flour mixture into the wet ingredients and then stir in carrots. Fill each muffin tin so that it is about ¾ full. Bake for 20 minutes or until fully cooked in the center (toothpick inserted will not have uncooked mix on it).

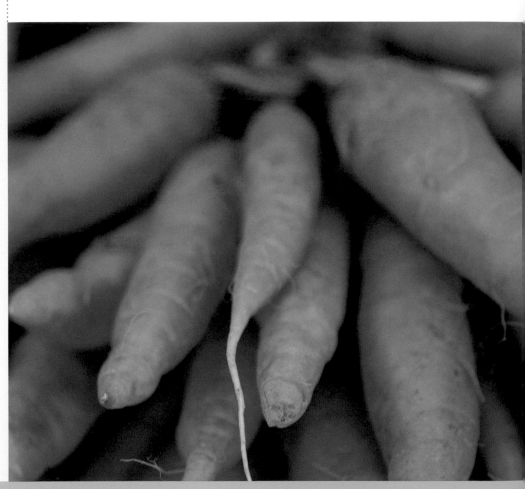

Visionary Muffins

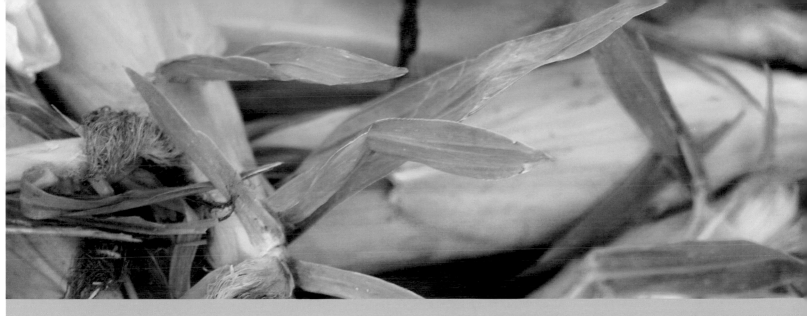

Copper Mountain Corn Bread

Preheat oven to 400°F. Lightly coat a 9 x 13" baking dish with cooking oil spray.

Whisk together eggs, melted butter, buttermilk, and whipping cream.

In a medium size bowl, stir together flour, corn meal, salt, sugar and baking powder.

Combine dry ingredients with wet ingredients and stir until just mixed. Be careful to not over-mix. Pour batter into prepared baking dish.

Bake for about 30 minutes. Serve warm with honey butter.

Per Serving:
228 Calories;
9g Fat (5g sat);
5g Protein;
34g Carbohydrate;
3g Dietary Fiber;
53mg Cholesterol;
294mg Sodium.

We make cornbread a lot when we're up skiing at Copper Mountain. It pairs perfectly with our Black Diamond Chili but goes with just about any soup there is. We choose to make this gluten-free version, which is more dense, but feel free to substitute whole wheat pastry flour for a cakier bread. Oh, and yes, it has a lot of butter, we know. If this concerns you feel free to substitute vegetable oil or try our Basic Cornbread Recipe. (next page)

Serves 20

3 eggs
8 tablespoons butter, melted
1½ cups lowfat buttermilk
½ cup whipping cream
2 cups brown rice flour
2 cups yellow corn meal
1½ teaspoons sea salt
¼ cup sugar
1 tablespoon baking powder

Maizy's Cornbread

Serves 12

1 cup lowfat milk
¼ cup canola oil
1 egg
¼ cup honey
1½ cups cornmeal
½ cup whole wheat flour
4 teaspoons baking powder
½ teaspoon sea salt

Per Serving:
197 Calories;
6g Fat (1 g sat);
4g Protein;
34g Carbohydrate;
3g Dietary Fiber;
19mg Cholesterol;
257mg Sodium.

Heat oven to 425°F. Grease bottom of 8 x 8 square pan.

Beat milk, oil, honey, and egg in medium-sized bowl. Stir in remaining ingredients all at once just until flour is moistened (batter will be lumpy).

Fill pan with batter. Bake until golden brown and toothpick inserted in center comes out clean, 20 to 25 minutes.

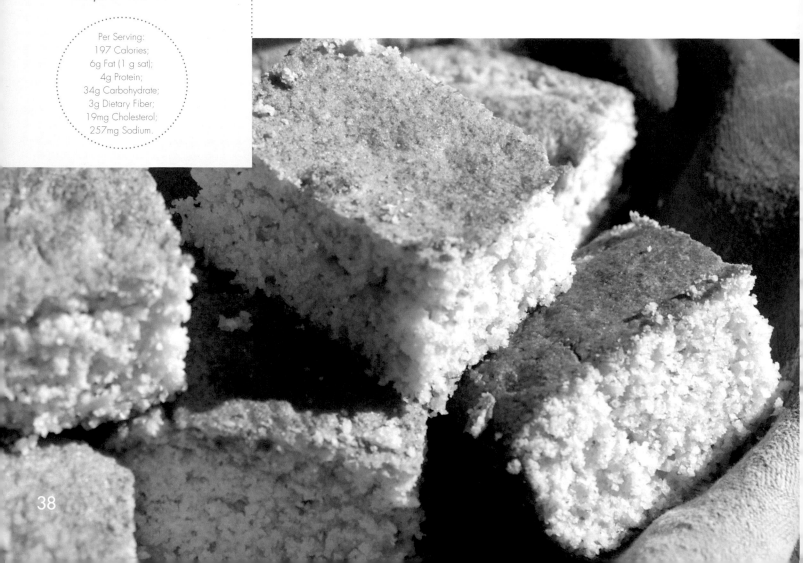

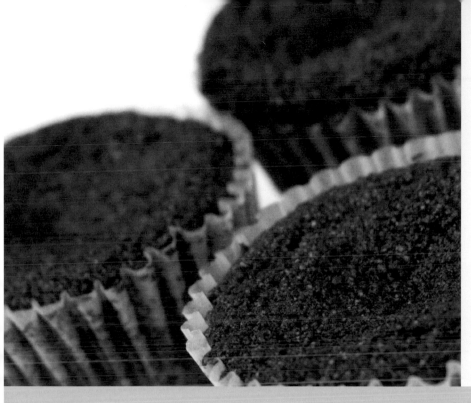

You are going to love the smell of these baking! These muffins are as nice on the breakfast or dinner table as they are served as dessert with a dollup of homemade whipped cream on the side. Molasses is actually a sweetener with some health benefits. Known mostly as an excellent source of iron, blackstrap molasses is also a good source of calcium.

Makes 12 muffins

Little Bear Peak Gingerbread Muffins

Heat oven to 400°F. Grease 12 medium muffin cups, or place paper baking cup in each muffin cup. Beat together brown sugar, molasses, milk, applesauce, and egg in a large bowl. In a separate bowl, whisk together flour through ground cloves. Stir dry ingredients into wet until just mixed.

Divide batter evenly among muffin cups. Bake 18 to 20 minutes or until toothpick inserted in center comes out clean. Immediately remove from pan to wire rack. Serve warm if desired.

¼ cup packed brown sugar
½ cup molasses
⅓ cup lowfat milk
⅓ cup applesauce, unsweetened
1 egg
2 cups whole wheat flour
1 teaspoon baking powder
1 teaspoon ground ginger
½ teaspoon salt
½ teaspoon baking soda
½ teaspoon ground cinnamon
¼ teaspoon ground cloves

Per Muffin
133 Calories;
1g Fat (trace sat);
3g Protein;
30g Carbohydrate;
3g Dietary Fiber;
16mg Cholesterol;
195mg Sodium.

Lemon-Ginger Muffins (Gluten Free)

Preheat oven to 375°F. Line a standard muffin tin with paper liners or coat evenly with cooking spray. If using a shallow muffin pan, this recipe will make closer to 16 muffins.

Cut the ginger into pieces and add to a food processor fitted with a metal blade. Process ginger until finely minced. You should have a heaping ¼ cup of fresh ginger. Add the ¼ cup of ginger, plus ¼ cup sugar in a small saucepan. Cook over medium heat until the sugar has melted, stirring constantly. This should take just a few minutes. Remove from heat. Stir in lemon zest and ¼ cup of sugar.

In a medium size bowl, whisk together flour, tapioca flour, cornmeal, baking powder and baking soda. Set aside.

In a large mixing bowl, beat butter until smooth. Add remaining ¼ cup of sugar and beat until well blended. Next add both eggs and beat. Add yogurt and beat again. Add dry ingredients to butter mixture and stir until blended. Stir in the ginger-lemon mixture.

Spoon batter into muffin tin cups until each one is about ¾ full. Bake for 20 to 25 minutes. Cool in the tins for a minute and then remove to wire rack to continue cooling.

If you love ginger like we do then you'll love these muffins. Perfect for a Sunday brunch, any time of the day and any time of the year.

Makes 12-16

3 ounces fresh ginger root
¾ cup sugar, divided
2 tablespoons grated lemon peel
1½ cups brown rice flour
½ cup tapioca flour**
¼ cup cornmeal
¾ teaspoon baking powder
¼ teaspoon baking soda
½ cup unsalted butter
2 eggs
1 cup plain yogurt

**If you can't find tapioca flour, you can substitute coconut flour, garfava flour or you can use 1¾ cups brown rice flour. As a non gluten-free alternative, feel free to substitute flour and cornmeal for 2 cups whole wheat pastry flour or all-purpose flour.

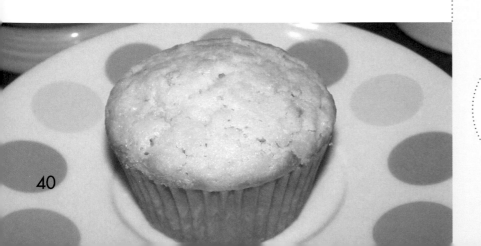

40

Per Serving:
189 Calories;
9g Fat (1g sat);
5g Protein;
25g Carbohydrate;
3g Dietary Fiber;
35mg Cholesterol;
140mg Sodium.

These muffins are surprisingly light and not too sweet, so don't be afraid to serve them at the dinner table. Well okay, we don't encourage chocolate chips at the dinner table, but as part of a Southwestern buffet, definitely. Afterall, cocoa and chocolate do contain some wonderful antioxidants that may benefit the heart and satisfy the soul.

Makes 18 muffins

¼ cup brewed decaffeinated coffee
½ cup lowfat 2% milk (can substitute soy milk or
   buttermilk)
½ cup canola (or other vegetable) oil
2 large eggs
1 teaspoon vanilla
1 ¾ cups whole wheat pastry flour
⅓ cup natural cane sugar
⅓ cup brown sugar
3 tablespoons cocoa powder
¾ teaspoon aluminum free baking powder
¾ teaspoon baking soda
1 pinch cayenne chili powder, about
⅛ teaspoon
¼ teaspoon salt
¾ cup semisweet chocolate chips
¾ cup pecans, coarsely chopped

Per Serving:
229 Calories;
14g Fat (4g sat);
4g Protein;
25g Carbohydrate;
3g Dietary Fiber;
24mg Cholesterol;
35mg Sodium.

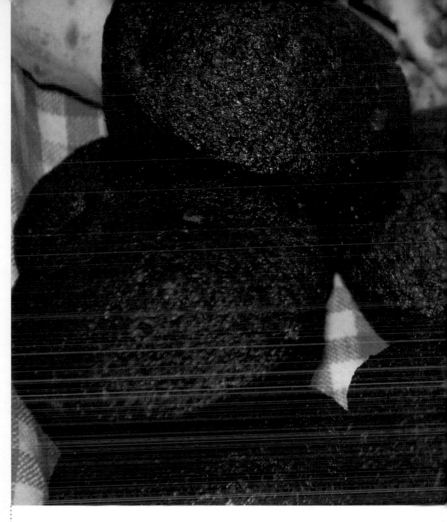

Preheat oven to 375°F. Line muffin tins with paper liners or cooking spray. In a medium bowl combine coffee, milk, oil, eggs, and vanilla and blend until mixed. In a large bowl combine flour, sugar, brown sugar, cocoa powder, baking powder, baking soda, cayenne, and salt. Stir to mix. Add wet ingredients to dry ingredients and stir until just combined. Stir in chocolate chips and pecans.

Fill muffin tins about half to three quarters full of batter. Bake about 20 minutes or until toothpick inserted into center of muffins comes out clean. Cool on wire rack.

M³ Muffins (Mucho Mocha Mole)

Pyramid Peak Pumpkin Bread

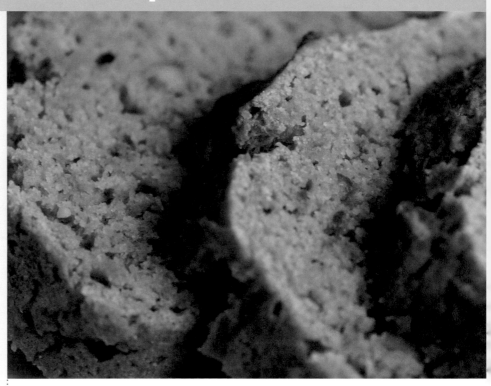

One-half a cup of canned pumpkin contains two and a half times the daily recommended requirement of beta-carotene, approximately 16 milligrams. Pumpkin is a great source of lutein and zeaxanthin, lesser-known carotenoids that protect the eye and may help block the formation of cataracts. Walnuts provide essential fats and fiber. Additional fiber is provided by the applesauce and whole wheat flour. A delicious holiday or anytime treat!

1 loaf (12 generous slices)

½ cup sugar
1 cup canned pumpkin
¼ cup canola oil
¼ cup applesauce
1 teaspoon vanilla extract
2 eggs
1 ¾ cups whole wheat flour
½ cup coarsely chopped walnuts
2 teaspoons baking powder
½ teaspoon ground cinnamon
¼ teaspoon salt
¼ teaspoon ground nutmeg
Cooking spray
parchment paper, optional

Per Serving:
189 Calories;
9g Fat (1g sat);
5g Protein;
25g Carbohydrate;
3g Dietary Fiber;
35mg Cholesterol;
140mg Sodium.

Heat oven to 350°F. Spray loaf pan lightly with cooking spray. Line bottom only with parchment paper.

In a large bowl, whisk together sugar, pumpkin, oil, applesauce, vanilla and eggs.

In another bowl stir together remaining ingredients (flour through nutmeg). Stir dry ingredients into the pumpkin mixture. Carefully pour into pan, using a spatula to scrape out any remaining batter from the bowl into the loaf pan.

Bake about 45 to 50 minutes, or until toothpick inserted in center comes out clean. Cool 10 minutes on a wire rack. Loosen sides of loaf from pan; remove from pan. Cool completely on wire rack before slicing. Store tightly wrapped in refrigerator up to 1 week or freeze.

Every summer when zucchini is most abundant, we bake up several batches of zucchini bread. There was a time when we liked to add protein powder to just about everything we baked including pancakes, muffins, even cookies. We don't do that quite as much these days, but we still add it to some of our baked goods to help balance out the carbohydrate load just a bit. Zucchini may not have the pronounced and celebrated health benefits as some of its close counterparts, but zucchini and summer squashes have been shown to have anti-cancer effects. They are a good source of vitamin C, manganese, magnesium, carotenoids (including beta-carotene), fiber, potassium, and folate.

Yield: 2 loaves (24 slices)

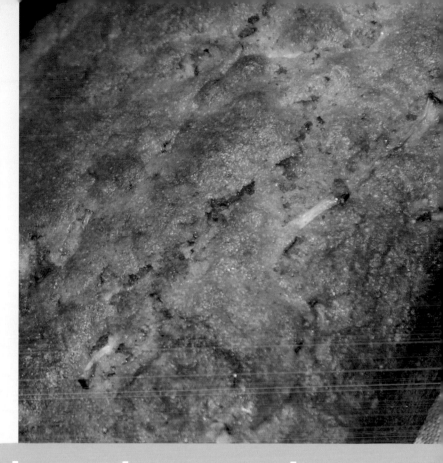

Jumpin' Jack Zucchini Bread

2½ cups shredded zucchini (about 3 medium)
1 cup sugar
⅓ cup canola oil
⅓ cup applesauce
1 teaspoon vanilla
4 eggs
2 ½ cups whole wheat flour
½ cup vanilla flavored whey protein powder (may substitute powdered milk or additional flour)
½ cup coarsely chopped walnuts or pecans
4 teaspoons baking powder
1 teaspoon salt
1 teaspoon ground cinnamon
½ teaspoon ground cloves

Heat oven to 350°F. Lightly coat 2 bread loaf pans with cooking spray. Whisk together zucchini, sugar, oil, applesauce, vanilla and eggs in a large bowl. In a separate bowl whisk together flour, protein powder, nuts, baking powder, salt, cinnamon, and cloves. Stir this dry mixture into the wet ingredients.

Bake 50 to 60 minutes (center rack) or until toothpick inserted in center comes out clean. Cool 10 minutes. Loosen sides of loaves from pans; remove from pans. Cool completely on wire rack before slicing. Store tightly wrapped in refrigerator up to 1 week.

Per Serving: (based on the addition of protein powder containing 12 grams protein per tablespoon): 134 Calories; 6g Fat (1g sat); 6g Protein; 19g Carbohydrate; 2g Dietary Fiber; 31mg Cholesterol, 181mg Sodium.

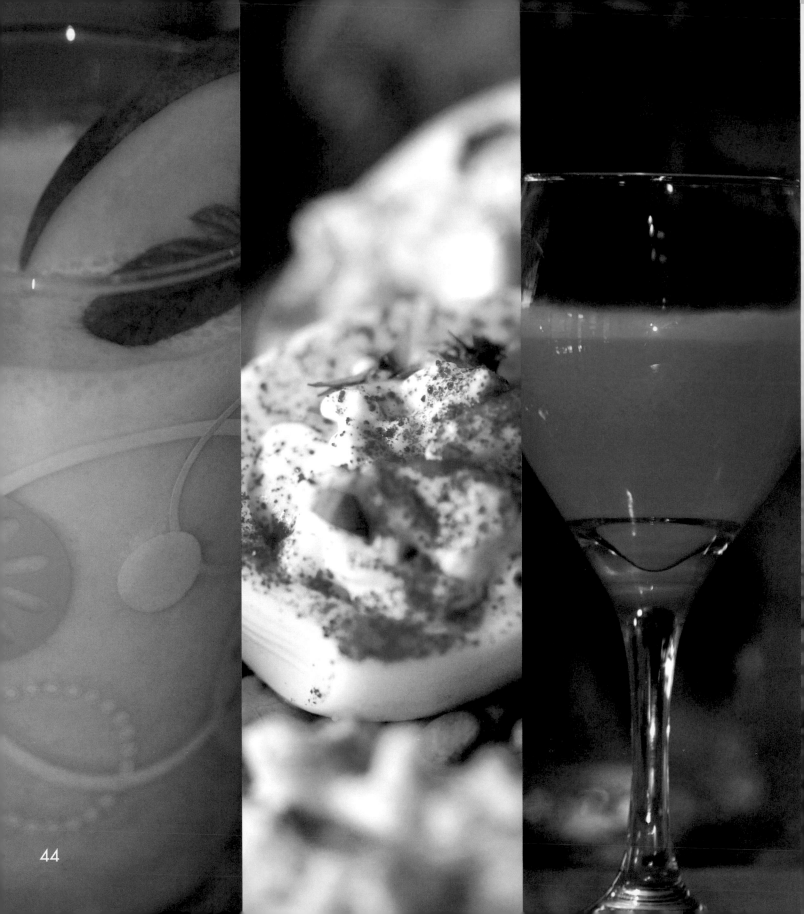

All that we are is the result of what we have thought. The mind is everything. What we think we become. ~Buddha

Power Boosts

Boosts

Healthy snacking may have become a lost art. There are just too many tempting high-calorie, low benefit, poor choices out there (that are just too easy to eat!) Strategic, smart snacking can be a great way to keep your energy going and your metabolism strong!

Look for snacks that are high in fiber, have at least 5 grams of protein and come in at around 200 calories. Here are some great and easy ideas:

- *Pear and slice of reduced fat Jarlsberg (Swiss) cheese*
- *Handful of almonds (about 10) and dried fruit (about ¼ cup)*
- *1 ounce of baked tortilla chips with ¼ cup of fat free refried beans, reduced fat cheese and salsa*
- *Fat-free Greek-style yogurt with low fat granola*
- *¼ cup Edamame (soybeans) with olive oil and a little black pepper*
- *½ cup cottage cheese with 5 grape tomatoes*
- *½ cup hummus on a rice cake or unlimited celery*
- *2 tablespoons peanut butter and ½ apple*
- *mix1*

These smarter snacks will help you achieve increased energy and metabolism!

The key to strategic snacking is to know when to stop. These tasty little squares are meant as a snack – that means just one.

Makes about 12 squares

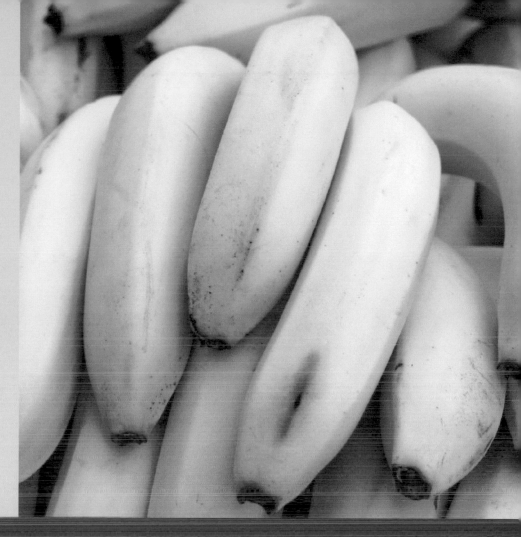

Peanut Butter Banana Squares

1 cup whole wheat flour
½ cup oats
¼ cup wheat germ
¼ cup ground flax seed
¼ cup brown sugar, packed
½ teaspoon baking soda
1 teaspoon baking powder
¼ teaspoon salt
1½ teaspoons cinnamon
1 cup lowfat milk
2 eggs
1 ripe banana, mashed
½ cup natural peanut butter

Preheat oven to 375°F. Lightly grease 8½" × 8½" square baking pan.

In a medium bowl, combine flour, oats, wheat germ, flax seed, sugar, baking soda, baking powder, salt, and cinnamon. Mix well. In another bowl, combine milk, eggs, banana and peanut butter. Add to dry ingredients. Bake for 25 to 35 minutes or until brown on top. Allow to cool about 10 minutes. Cut into 12 bars.

Per Serving:
209 Calories;
9g Fat (1g sat);
8g Protein;
24g Carbohydrate;
4g Dietary Fiber;
35mg Cholesterol;
197mg Sodium.

47

These bars are full of essential omega-3 fatty acids and a good source of protein and balanced complex carbohydrates. If you have a food dehydrator, you can mix together all the ingredients and spread on a dehydrator sheet. For a totally "raw" experience, omit the protein powder and chocolate chips – instead you can add a few cacao nibs.

Makes 15 bars

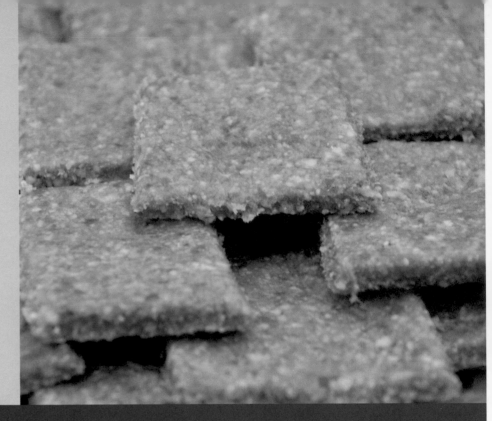

Balanced Energy Bars ("BE" Bars)

½ cup Brazil nuts
½ cup walnuts
¼ cup ground flax seed
¼ cup hemp seeds (also referred to as hemp nuts)
½ cup pumpkin seeds
1 scoop whey protein powder
¼ teaspoon ground cinnamon
¼ cup organic almond butter
12 dates, pitted
¼ cup agave nectar (or honey)
¼ cup organic chocolate chips

Per Bar:
188 Calories;
12g Fat (2g sat);
7g Protein;
16g Carbohydrate;
3g Dietary Fiber;
1mg Cholesterol;
7mg Sodium

Line an 8 x 13 baking dish with parchment paper.

Combine Brazil nuts through ground cinnamon in bowl of food processor fitted with steel blade. Process until the nuts are finely ground. Add almond butter, dates, and agave nectar (or honey) and process until mixture starts to stick together. Add chocolate chips and pulse until evenly distributed.

Using a wooden spoon or your clean hands, press ground nut mixture into prepared baking dish. Cover with foil or wrap and refrigerate for at least an hour before slicing. To retain freshness, refrigerate and store in air-tight container.

48

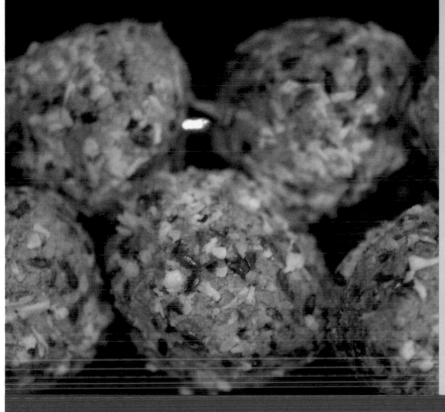

This recipe is easily adaptable according to your mood or dietary restrictions. Here is a basic recipe. These snack "balls" are similar to the BE bars, just in a rounder format. You can interchange nuts, seeds, nut butters, protein powder, and sweetener. This is a guideline. Again the protein powder is optional.

Makes 16

Perfect Power Snack Balls

Mix all ingredients together in large bowl. Mixture should be somewhat tacky but not "wet." If it seems too moist to work with, add more protein powder or more ground nuts. Take 1 to 2 tablespoons of the mixture and roll it into a ball and place it on a cookie sheet or other relatively flat surface. You can roll the balls in dried coconut or chopped nuts. You can eat right away or refrigerate for a firmer snack. Store in an airtight container in the refrigerator.

⅓ cup ground almonds
⅓ cup ground pumpkin seeds
⅓ cup ground flax seed
⅓ cup peanut butter
⅓ cup sesame tahini
3 tablespoons maple syrup
⅓ cup protein powder

Other options:
Organic dried fruit such as currants, dates, or raisins
Organic dried, flaked coconut

Per Serving:
129 Calories;
8g Fat (1g sat);
8g Protein;
8g Carbohydrate;
2g Dietary Fiber;
2mg Cholesterol;
44mg Sodium.

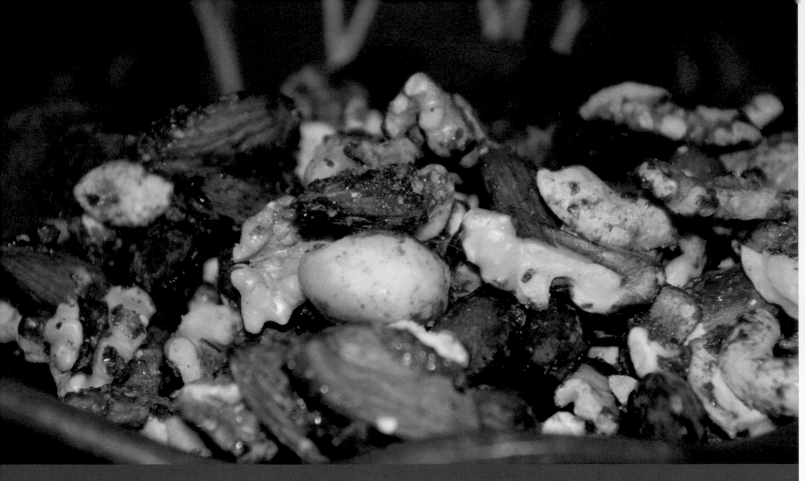

Sweet and Spicy Nuts

Combine sugar, pepper, and spices in a small bowl and mix well. Heat a large frying pan or cast iron skillet over medium high and add the nuts. Sprinkle the spice mixture over the nuts and stir frequently over medium heat for about 5 minutes or until the nuts start to turn golden and the sugar begins to caramelize. Once the sugar has fully dissolved and caramelized, remove from heat and spread nuts on a piece of parchment or aluminum foil, in a single layer, until they have completely cooled.

Per Serving:
219 Calories;
18g Fat (1g sat);
7g Protein;
11g Carbohydrate;
3g Dietary Fiber;
0mg Cholesterol;
136mg Sodium

Serves 6 to 8

2 cups mixed raw nuts (almonds,walnuts, cashews, pecans, macadamia nuts)
3 tablespoons sugar
½ teaspoon ground black pepper
1 teaspoon cinnamon
½ teaspoon curry powder, Can also substitute Cajun seasoning
1 pinch ground cloves
¼ teaspoon ground cumin

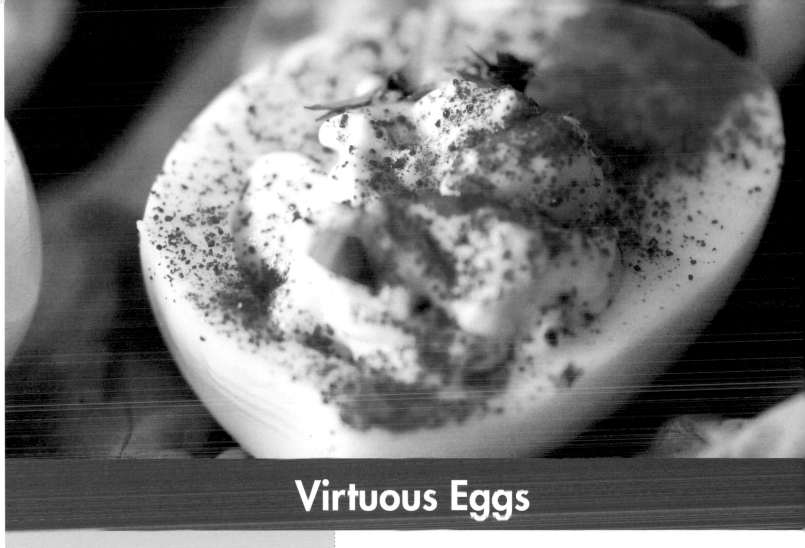

Virtuous Eggs

Serves 6

6 hard-cooked eggs, peeled
2 tablespoons plain yogurt
2 tablespoons lowfat cottage cheese
1 tablespoon finely chopped green onion
1 teaspoon mustard
¼ teaspoon sea salt
¼ teaspoon of dried dill
1 teaspoon horseradish
½ teaspoon paprika
1 teaspoon fresh parsley, finely chopped

Cut eggs lengthwise in half. Slip out egg yolks; mash with fork. Whisk in yogurt, cottage cheese, green onion, mustard, salt, dill and horseradish. If you want a smoother texture then feel free to use an electric beater or blender. Fill egg white halves with egg yolk mixture, heaping slightly. You can either do this simply with a spoon or get fancy using a pastry bag fitted with the piping tip. Garnish with paprika and parsley.

Other fun hard boiled egg fillings:
Hummus
Guacamole
Roasted Red Pepper Spread
Baba Gannoush

Per Serving
(2 halves): 83 Calories;
5g Fat (2g sat);
7g Protein;
1g Carbohydrate;
trace Dietary Fiber;
212mg Cholesterol;
164mg Sodium.

Body-Boosting Beverages

Smoothies are growing in popularity and hard to resist…they are creamy and delicious. These days they come ready-to-eat, super-sized, and equipped with seductive names and sexy packaging! They have always been a "fave" for the health zealots but it appears smoothies have gone mainstream! And that isn't necessarily a good thing – some of the commercial "smoothies" pack more sugar than a milk shake.

To ensure the health benefits of a smoothie or a juice, it's best to make your own. To decrease the sugar load in the smoothie, use yogurt, nut or seed milk instead of fruit juice and add fresh or frozen fruit in place of the juice.

Adding powdered greens and other superfoods can really boost your daily antioxidant consumption. They are delicious and do not add many calories or sugar!

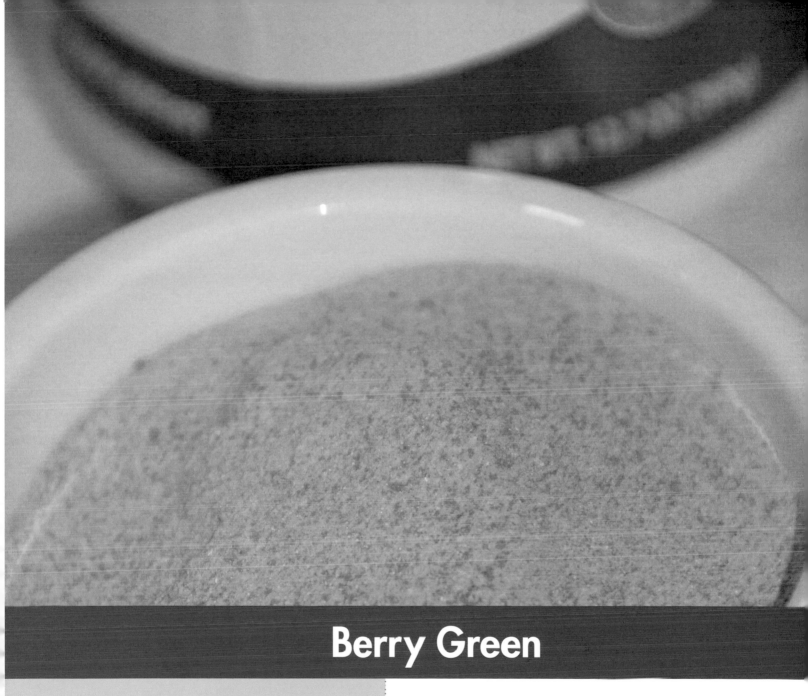

Berry Green

Serves 2 (tall glasses)

2 tablespoons organic whey protein powder
2 cups organic frozen raspberries or strawberries
1 cup plain or vanilla low-fat yogurt
1 cup lowfat milk
2 tablespoons greens
Optional: Ice cubes

In a blender, combine all the
ingredients and blend until smooth.
Pour into 2 glasses and serve cold.
Add water to thin.

Per Serving:
403 Calories;
5g Fat (1g sat);
12g Protein;
83g Carbohydrate;
13g Dietary Fiber;
7mg Cholesterol;
196mg Sodium.

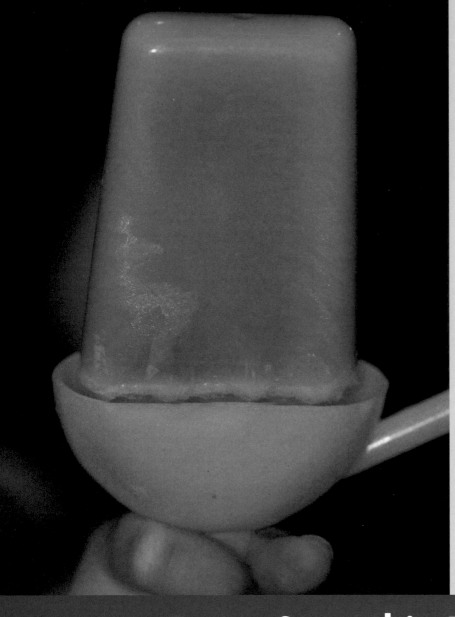

We always keep a batch of healthy popsicles on hand. You can use any one of the smoothie recipes in the book – or we also like mix1 popsicles.

Serves 4

Per Serving:
92 Calories;
1g Fat (1g sat);
6g Protein;
15g Carbohydrate;
1g Dietary Fiber;
6mg Cholesterol;
76mg Sodium.

Berry Smoothie Popsicles

Place yogurt, milk, strawberries, and banana in blender or food processor. Add 2 tablespoons of your favorite vanilla protein powder. Pulse or blend for a few more seconds to fully incorporate the protein powder. Cover and blend on high speed about 30 seconds or until smooth.

Add smoothie mixture to popsicle forms. Freeze at least 2 hours or until solid enough to remove from form. Drink any leftovers!

Plastic popsicle forms (available at most grocery stores or kitchen stores)
1 cup plain nonfat or lowfat yogurt
1 cup lowfat milk
½ cup fresh or frozen strawberries
½ cup fresh or frozen blueberries
½ banana
2 tablespoons protein powder

This is a warming tea that may help improve digestion. The flavor is reminiscent of chai tea. Perfect for a cold winter day.

Serves 2

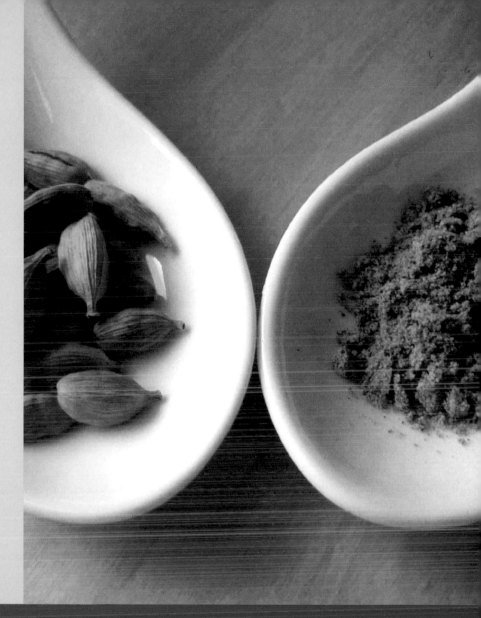

Per Serving:
32 Calories;
trace Fat (0g sat);
1g Protein;
7g Carbohydrate;
trace Dietary Fiber;
1mg Cholesterol;
19mg Sodium.

Cardamom Ginger Tea

1 tablespoon fresh ginger, sliced
1 teaspoon cardamom seeds
1 cinnamon stick, broken in a few pieces
3 cups of water
1 tablespoon agave nectar (or honey)
2 tablespoons of 2% milk

In a small saucepan, combine 1 tablespoon fresh ginger, cardamom seeds, and cinnamon stick pieces plus 3 cups of water. Bring water to a boil, then reduce heat and continue to simmer for about 5 to 10 minutes. Turn off heat and stir in agave nectar or honey. Strain solids from tea and pour tea into a teapot. Stir in 2 tablespoons of milk. Serve immediately.

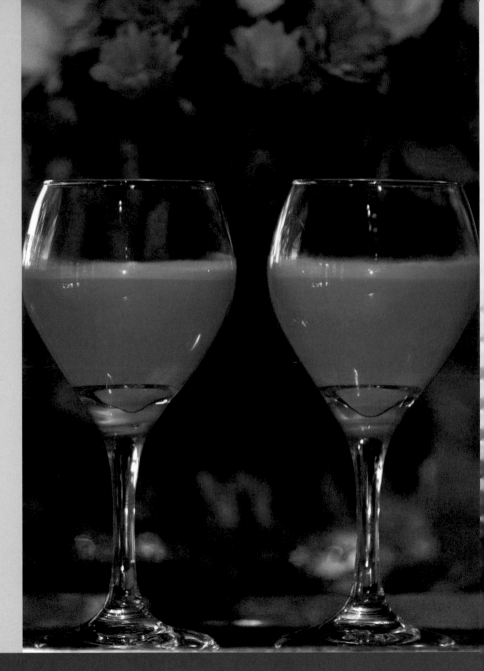

You really need a juicer or a Vitamix blender to successfully navigate this juice. Super-refreshing and energizing, this is also a nice cleansing juice. One advantage of this juice includes glowing skin.

Serves 2

Per Serving:
92 Calories;
1g Fat (1g sat);
6g Protein;
15g Carbohydrate;
1g Dietary Fiber;
6mg Cholesterol;
76mg Sodium.

Carrot, Apple, Lemon, Ginger Juice

6 medium carrots, washed and sliced
1 medium size apple, washed and quartered
2 inches ginger, about 3 tablespoons
½ small lemon

Wash vegetables well. Slice them so that they can fit into the feeding area of your juicer. With most juicers there is no need to remove seeds or peels prior to juicing. Juice into tall glass or mason jar. When finished juicing, stir to combine and enjoy right away.

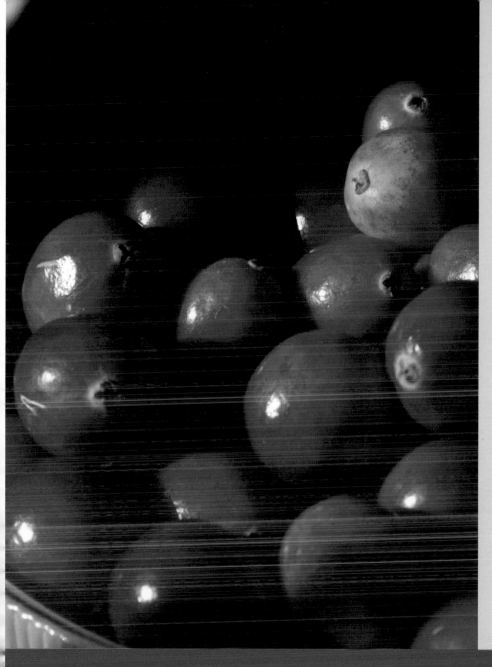

You can feel good about serving this non-alcoholic version of a mimosa at any brunch or party. To turn it into a wine "cooler" you can add the juice mixture to about 8 ounces of white wine — for a wine spritzer, you can add wine (about 9 ounces) to the recipe as it exists and call it good for 3 people. There are definitely great things to say about cranberry juice — and in the unsweetened form it sure can do wonders for a urinary tract infection — however we wouldn't recommend this recipe to anyone with a current UTI, due to the higher sugar content of the nectar plus other juices.

Serves 2

Per Serving:
132 Calories;
trace Fat (0 sat);
1g Protein;
32g Carbohydrate;
trace Dietary Fiber;
0mg Cholesterol;
5mg Sodium.

Citrus Cranberry Mocktail

Combine orange juice, pineapple juice and cranberry nectar juice in a blender or you can stir them together in a small pitcher. Add mineral water and stir once again to combine. Pour into two white wine glasses or juice glasses and garnish with an orange slice.

½ cup fresh squeezed orange juice
¼ cup pineapple juice
½ cup cranberry nectar juice
  (We like Santa Cruz Organics)
1 cup mineral water, chilled
Orange slices (optional for garnish)

57

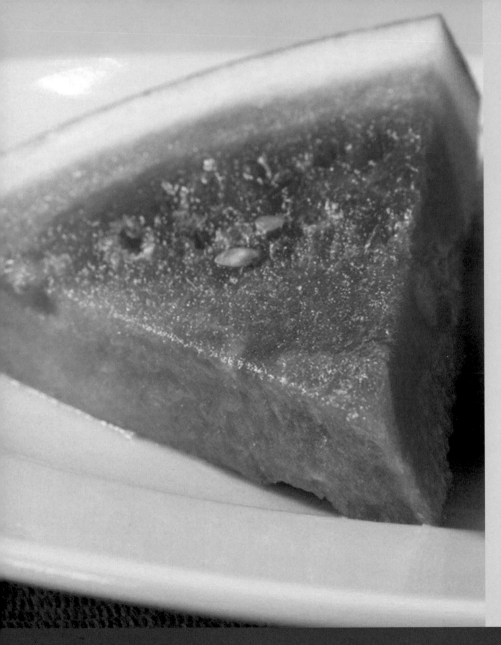

This juice has wonderful cleansing and supportive nutrients for the kidneys and bladder.

Serves 2

Per Serving:
189 Calories;
2g Fat (trace sat);
2g Protein;
44g Carbohydrate;
2g Dietary Fiber;
0mg Cholesterol;
10mg Sodium.

Kidney Cleanser

Add all ingredients to juicer and juice into one glass or mason jar. Alternatively you can add ½ cup apple juice plus pineapple and watermelon to a blender – but cut the watermelon to 1 cup in this case.

2 apples
1 cup pineapple cubes
2 cups seedless watermelon

If you haven't tried any of the coconut milk ice cream or yogurt that is out now, we encourage you to do so – it is extremely fabulous. Turtle Mountain's Purely Decadent frozen desserts are amazing. The added protein only adds to the light fluffiness of this shake, rather than weighing it down – plus the protein balances the carbohydrate hit so you won't bonk like you would after drinking a regular "conventional" milkshake. For a thinner shake you can add less ice, a little water or more almond "milk."

Serves 1

Per Serving:
393 Calories;
15g Fat (11g sat);
27g Protein;
43g Carbohydrate;
9g Dietary Fiber;
0mg Cholesterol;
260mg Sodium.

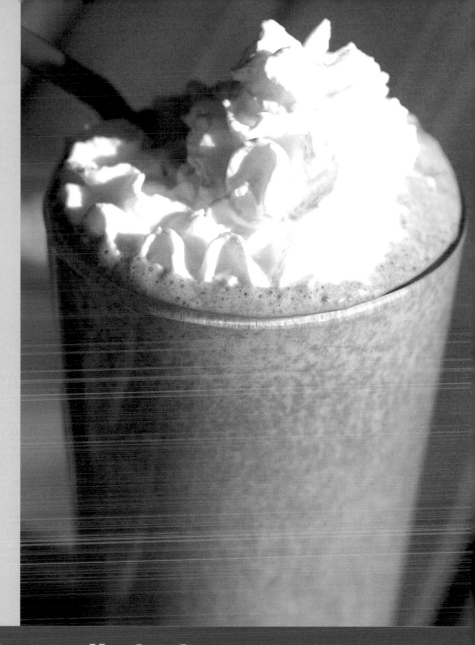

Mock "Milkshake"

½ cup chocolate coconut milk ice cream
¾ cup chocolate almond milk
1 scoop chocolate whey protein powder
ice cubes

Add all of the ingredients to a blender and blend until smooth. Add ice cubes to adjust thickness to desired liking.

We tend to add protein powder to most of our smoothies to balance out the sugars, but this is always optional. We spent many days picking blackberries in Oregon – sometimes they're sour, sometimes they're sweet, but they are always packed with phytonutrients, vitamins, minerals, and antioxidants.

Serves 2

Per Serving:
156 Calories;
2g Fat (trace sat);
10g Protein;
26g Carbohydrate;
5g Dietary Fiber;
5mg Cholesterol;
47mg Sodium.

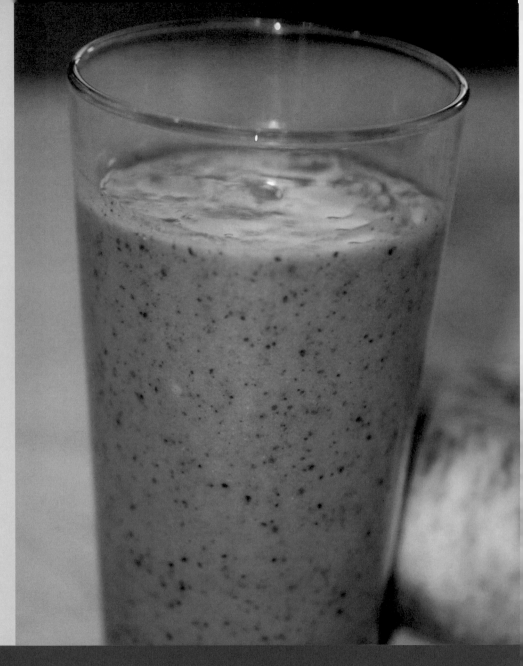

Summer Daze

1 cup fresh or frozen blackberries
½ cup peach nectar
½ cup lowfat milk of choice
¼ cup lowfat vanilla yogurt
1 cup crushed ice (approximate)
1 tablespoon vanilla protein powder

Add all of the ingredients except protein powder to a blender. Purée on high for about 20 seconds – you may need to use the "ice crush" button as well. Add a tablespoon of your favorite vanilla protein powder. Pulse or blend for a few more seconds to fully incorporate the protein powder.

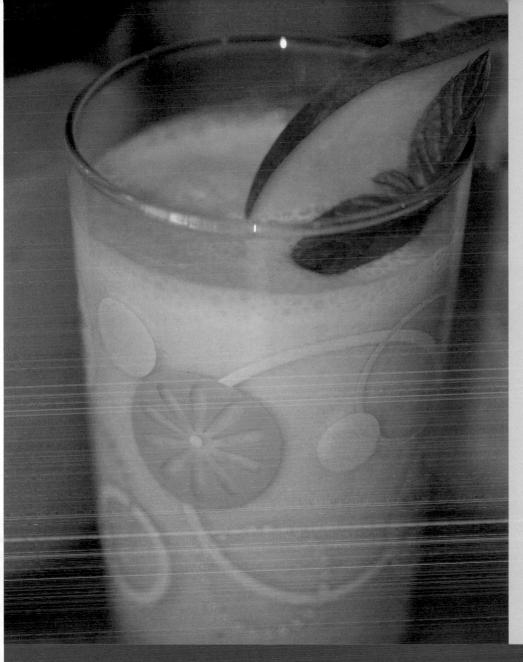

This smoothie is loaded with flavor, fiber and packed with vitamin C. This is a nice mid-morning pick-me-up or breakfast substitute. If you use frozen papaya then it will be a little thicker. The tropical nature of this smoothie is a real treat. If you know that you don't have sensitivity to berries, then strawberries are a great addition to this smoothie. The rice protein powder is suitable for vegetarians and anyone with sensitivity to soy or dairy-based protein powders.

Serves 2

Per Serving (may differ depending on type of protein powder used). 185 Calories; trace Fat; (trace sat), 3g Protein; 44g Carbohydrate; 4g Dietary Fiber; 1mg Cholesterol; 205mg Sodium

Tropical Treasure

Add all ingredients to blender and blend until smooth.

1 cup pineapple juice
½ cup guava juice
½ papaya, seeded and peeled
1 cup ice cubes
4 tablespoons whey or rice protein powder, vanilla

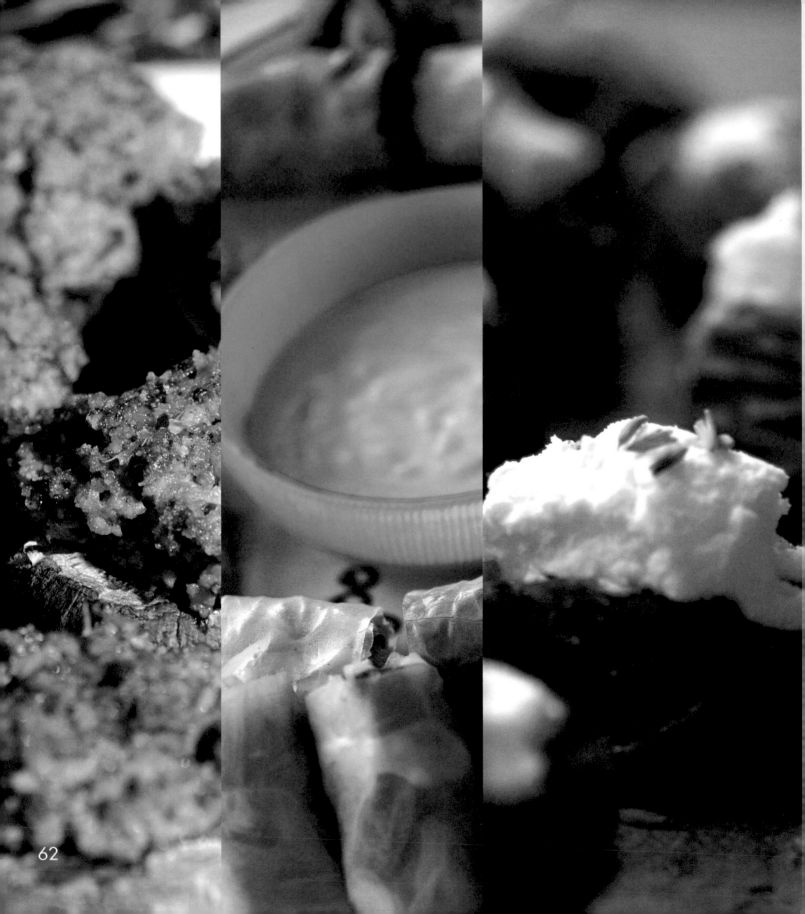

It's so beautifully arranged on the plate - you know someone's fingers have been all over it. ~ Julia Child

Modest Bites

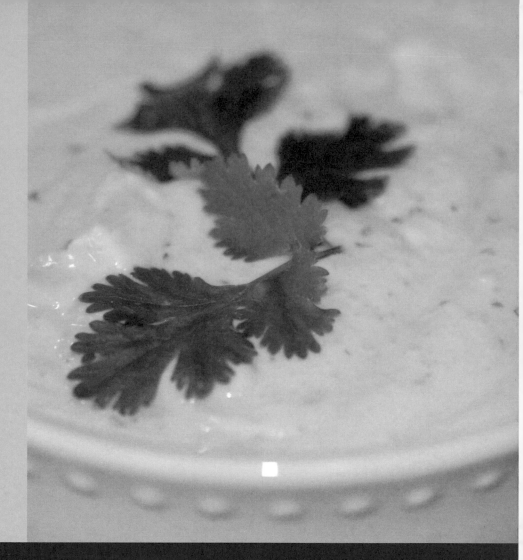

This is actually a much lighter version of your standard guacamole. You'll love the creaminess. Serve with raw veggies or veggie chips.

(Yields about 3 cups) Serves 6 to 10

Per Serving:
136 Calories;
9g Fat (1g sat);
7g Protein;
10g Carbohydrate;
2g Dietary Fiber;
4mg Cholesterol;
45mg Sodium.

Almost Guacamole

1 cup plain nonfat yogurt (Greek-style)
1 cup nonfat sour cream
2 avocados, peeled, pitted and halved
1 clove garlic, minced
2 tablespoons finely chopped fresh cilantro
½ teaspoon ground cumin
1 tablespoon lime or lemon juice
1 teaspoon jalapeno pepper, seeded and minced
salt and pepper, if desired

Combine yogurt, sour cream and avocado in the bowl of a food processor fitted with the blade attachment. Add remaining ingredients. Process and purée until smooth. Cover and refrigerate at least 1 hour to blend flavors.

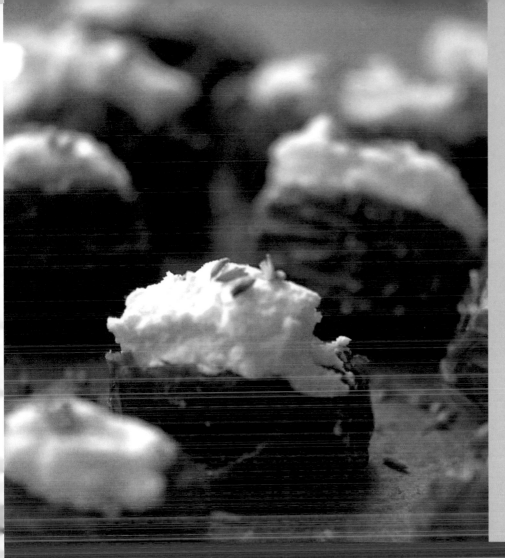

Even if you're not a big chevre fan, this bite-sized appetizer is a palate pleaser. Dates are rich in fiber, magnesium, iron, and calcium — just to name a few of the many nutrients found in dates. The lavender flowers give this modest bite a summery feel.

Serves 8

Per Serving:
(1 date)103 Calories;
6g Fat (4g sat);
4g Protein;
8g Carbohydrate;
1g Dietary Fiber;
17mg Cholesterol,
109mg Sodium.

Stuffed Dates with Chevre and Lavender

Remove the pit from each date so that there forms a gaping opening. In a small-medium size bowl, blend together Neufchatel, chevre, lavender and honey. Spoon about a teaspoon of the cheese mixture into the center of the date. Garnish with fresh lavender flowers or sprigs as desired.

For an added extravagance, wrap each date with prosciutto.

8 dates, pitted
¼ cup Neufchatel cheese
4 ounces chevre cheese
1 teaspoon fresh lavender flowers
1 tablespoon honey or agave nectar

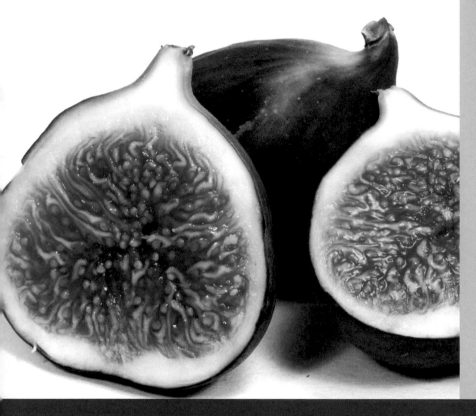

Fresh figs are really only available during the summer months. They are loaded with fiber and potassium. These are "off the charts" and gluten-free.

Serves 4

Fig Quesadillas

Preheat oven to 350°F. Prepare large baking sheet by spraying with olive oil spray. Place tortillas on the baking sheet 2 at a time. Spread ¼ cup of cheese on the bottom half of each tortilla. Add a layer of fig, distributing evenly. Sprinkle each with some red onion, cilantro, and green chili sauce. Top each with another ¼ cup of cheese. Fold the tortillas over to make half circles and press down lightly.

Bake 8 minutes on each side, so that each side is lightly browned. Remove pan from oven and cool slightly. Transfer to cutting board and cut into 2 or 4 wedges each.

4 Brown Rice Tortillas (if you can't find these you can use regular flour tortillas)
2 cups grated cheddar and/or jack cheese
1½ cups diced fresh figs
2 tablespoons diced red onion
2 tablespoons minced cilantro
2 tablespoons green chili sauce
olive oil spray

Per Serving:
431 Calories;
23g Fat (13g sat);
19g Protein; 43g
Carbohydrate;
5g Dietary Fiber;
59mg Cholesterol;
736mg Sodium.

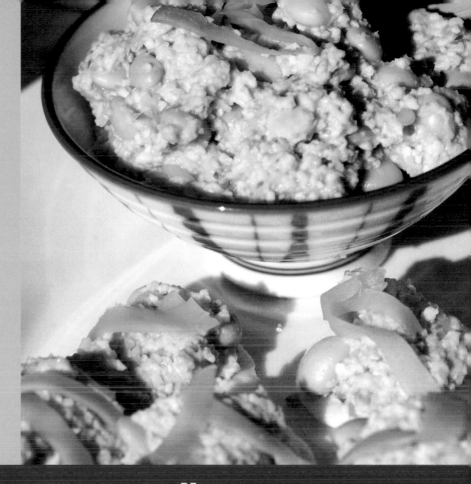

We were inspired by this recipe when one of our magazine partners at Vegetarian Times came out with it. James featured it on 9news and had a ton of positive feedback on it so we decided to include it here. Edamame is a terrific protein source for vegetarians. Choose organic edamame whenever possible since soy, like corn, is one of the most genetically modified crops across the globe.

Serves 12

Me Soy Tasty Tidbits

1 16-oz. pkg. frozen shelled edamame
1 cup thinly sliced green onions (about
  2 bunches)
2 tablespoons, red or yellow miso
24 slices pickled ginger, plus 2 Tbs. juice
24 rice crackers

Per Serving:
79 Calories;
2.5g Fat (.5g sat);
5g Protein;
9g Carbohydrate;
2g Dietary Fiber;
0mg Cholesterol;
240mg Sodium.

Cook edamame according to package directions. Drain, and reserve ½ cup cooking water. Place 1 cup cooked edamame, ½ cup green onions, miso, ginger juice and reserved cooking water in bowl of food processor. Purée until smooth. Transfer to bowl, and stir in remaining edamame and green onions. Cover with plastic wrap, and chill until ready to assemble. Can be stored up to 24 hours.

Spoon 2 teaspoons edamame mixture onto each rice cracker. Top with ginger slices, and serve.

We will admit right here and now that these can be messy in the making and the cooking. Be prepared for a little splatter and know that it is well worth it in the end - just be sure to wear an apron while you're cooking these little morsels! We started making these when we lived in Albuquerque, New Mexico – a brief, yet significant time in our lives.

Makes 8 to 10

Per Serving:
123 Calories;
4g Fat (1g sat);
11g Protein;
10g Carbohydrate;
1g Dietary Fiber;
62mg Cholesterol;
273mg Sodium.

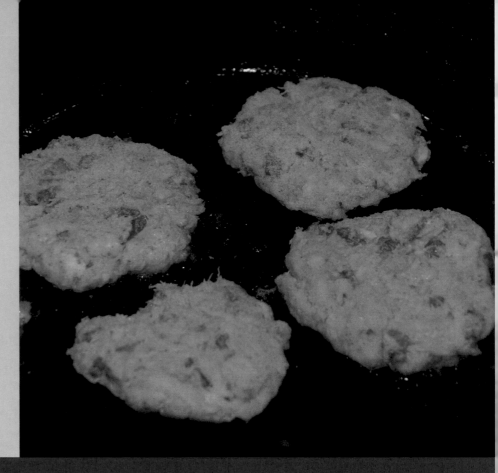

Sangre de Cristo Crab Cakes

1 tablespoon butter
¼ cup red bell pepper, minced
¼ cup celery, minced
1½ teaspoons jalapeno chile pepper,
* seeded and minced*
¼ cup lowfat mayonnaise
1 teaspoon dijon mustard
1 tablespoon fresh cilantro
1 egg, slightly beaten
1 teaspoon garlic powder
¼ teaspoon black pepper
¼ cup green onion
1 pound lump crabmeat
¾ cup bread crumbs
1 cup corn kernels
Cooking oil spray

Preheat oven to 450°F. Melt butter in small sauce pan. Add red bell pepper, celery and jalapeno and sauté for about 4 minutes and remove from heat.

In a medium to large size bowl, combine mayonnaise and next 7 ingredients. Mix well. Stir in bread crumbs and corn kernels. Add sautéed peppers and celery, mix well.

Form mixture into 10 equal size patties. Pan sear each patty in a cast-iron skillet coated with olive oil cooking spray. Flip each patty over and carefully move to the oven (be sure to wear an oven mitt when you move these) and bake for an additional 6 minutes. Serve warm with salsa or your topping of choice.

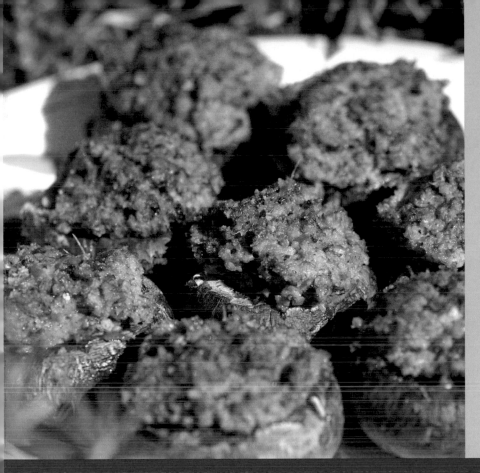

Cremini mushrooms have an impressive amount of nutrients ranging from minerals like selenium, copper, potassium, phosphorus, zinc, and manganese, to vitamins like B2 (riboflavin), B3 (niacin), B5 (pantothenic acid), B6 (pyridoxine), fiber, protein, and a fairly high amount of tryptophan. They also contain anticancer phytonutrients.

Serves 4

Per Serving:
79 Calories;
5g Fat (1g sat);
3g Protein;
6g Carbohydrate;
1g Dietary Fiber;
2mg Cholesterol;
83mg Sodium.

Pesto-Stuffed Mushrooms

Preheat oven to 350°F (unless making ahead). Heat oil in a nonstick skillet over medium heat. Add mushroom stems, and cook 5 minutes, stirring often. Break sausage into small pieces, add to skillet and brown 10 minutes, stirring often. Transfer mixture to food processor and pulse to chop. Add breadcrumbs and pesto, and pulse until just combined. Season with salt and pepper. Stuff into mushrooms, slightly mounding tops.

Arrange mushrooms in 9x9-inch ungreased baking dish. (If making ahead, cover with foil, and refrigerate.) Add ¼ cup water to dish, tightly cover with foil and bake 10 minutes. Remove foil, and bake 5 minutes more, or until browned. Serve hot.

Prepared pesto makes these mushrooms super-easy to assemble. To make ahead, stuff the mushrooms the day before, refrigerate, then pop them in the oven 20 minutes before you're ready to serve.

1 teaspoon olive oil
8 medium-sized cremini mushrooms,
  stems removed and chopped
2 oz. (¼ cup) ground sausage, (chicken, pork
  or soy)
2 tablespoons breadcrumbs
2 tablespoons pesto
salt and pepper to taste

Shrimp Spring Rolls with Peanut Sauce

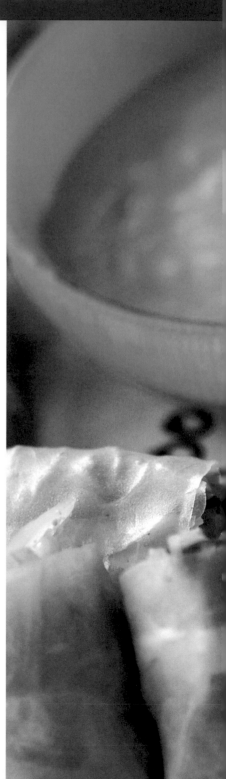

Prepare peanut sauce by combining all ingredients (except water) in a food processor or blender. Add water a little bit at a time until smooth and desired consistency is reached.

Rinse, peel and devein shrimp. Pat dry with paper towels and then chop the shrimp into smaller pieces (about ¾ inches long).

In a wok or skillet, heat grapeseed oil over high heat. Add shrimp and ⅛ teaspoon of salt, stir-fry for a minute or two until shrimp is cooked through. Remove shrimp from heat and set aside again in a bowl. Heat the wok or skillet again to medium high and add onions (or shallots) and ginger. Stir-fry about a minute and then add zucchini. Stir-fry the zucchini about 3 minutes then add fish sauce, tamari, broth and saute another 2 minutes. Add cabbage and sauté an additional minute.

Drain zucchini mixture and combine it with shrimp. Allow to cool.

Clear a clean spot on your kitchen counter or cutting board.

Fill a pie dish with very hot tap water. Place one tapioca or rice paper spring roll at a time in the hot water and wait until it softens, about 30 seconds. Remove from the water and place on your clean surface. Blot any excess water from the spring roll with a clean dish towel.

Toward the bottom of the spring roll place one lettuce leaf. Top with 1 tablespoon of the peanut sauce. Place 2 basil leaves on top of the peanut sauce. Add a few tablespoons of the zucchini and shrimp mixture (space it out so that you have about 4 shrimp laying flat and spaced evenly over the basil). Starting with the sides of the wrapper, gently fold over about ½ inch of the wrapper over the contents then roll up from one end to the other, keeping the roll tight like an egg roll or sushi roll. You ideally want to form a tightly compacted roll. Serve whole or cut in half.

Serving size is one roll for an appetizer and two rolls for a meal. Enjoy with sliced mango or papaya.

Per Serving:
(each roll)
192 Calories; 9g Fat
(2g sat); 14g Protein;
10g Carbohydrate;
4g Dietary Fiber;
65mg Cholesterol;
188mg Sodium.

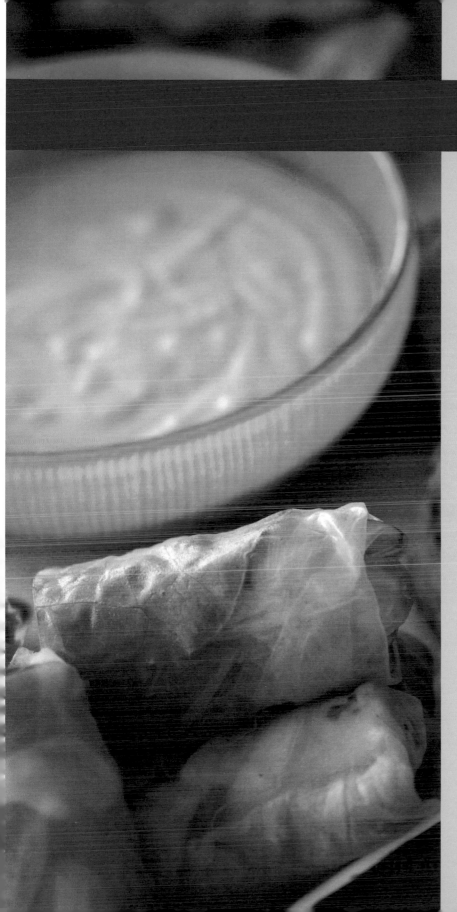

Making spring rolls can seem daunting at first but once you have all the ingredients layed out and ready to go, these roll up in a snap and are a real crowd pleaser.

Serves 4 to 8

Peanut Sauce:
½ cup peanut butter
¼ medium jalapeno chile pepper, seeded and chopped
1 garlic clove, minced
1 tablespoon chili sauce
1 teaspoon fish sauce
1 teaspoon hoisin sauce
1 teaspoon rice wine vinegar
1 tablespoon lemon juice, or lime juice
½ cup water

Rolls:
¾ pound shrimp, peeled and deveined
⅛ teaspoon of salt
⅛ teaspoon grapeseed oil or canola oil
½ small onion
1 tablespoon fresh ginger, minced
1 zucchini cut into matchsticks
½ teaspoon fish sauce
½ teaspoon tamari soy sauce
¼ cup low sodium vegetable broth
1 cup Chinese (or Napa) cabbage, shredded
8 lettuce leaves
16 basil leaves
8 spring roll wrappers (rice paper or tapioca)

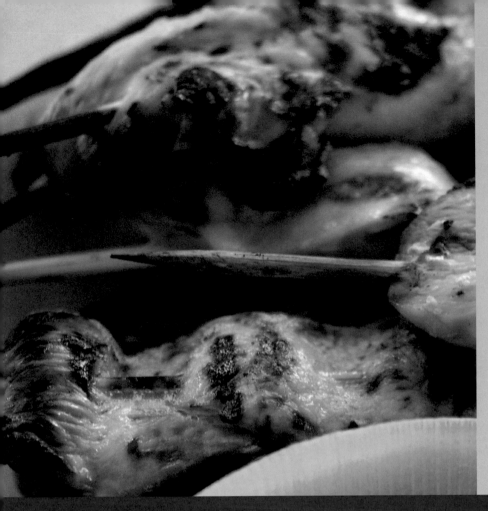

This is a standard at most of our larger gatherings. If we know vegetarians will be attending, we'll make extra vegetable skewers as well.

Serves 4

Per Serving:
183 Calories;
1g Fat (trace sat);
27g Protein;
15g Carbohydrate;
trace Dietary Fiber;
66mg Cholesterol;
525mg Sodium.

Skewered Teriyaki Chicken

Combine soy sauce, white wine vinegar, garlic, ginger, honey and onion powder in a medium size bowl. Add chicken pieces, cover and marinate in refrigerator for about 2 hours.

Soak wooden skewers in water for at least 20 minutes prior to threading on chicken. Preheat grill to medium high heat. Thread chicken onto skewers so that the chicken is evenly distributed. Grill over medium high heat for about 4 minutes and then flip and grill another few minutes until the chicken is cooked through with no pink spots.

Serve with spicy peanut sauce.

3 tablespoons wheat free tamari soy sauce or Bragg's Liquid Aminos
2 tablespoons white wine or rice vinegar
1 teaspoon minced garlic
1 teaspoon minced ginger
3 tablespoons honey or agave
¼ teaspoon onion powder
1 pound skinless boneless chicken breast cut into 2 inch pieces
8 wooden skewers or metal skewers

We first discovered this recipe in Cooking Light magazine. We changed a few of the ingredients and have served variations of this wonderful appetizer many times. You can experiment with different types of lettuces – radicchio is one option. You can also skip the lettuce and orange sections, and serve this on top of sliced heirloom tomatoes.

Serves 8

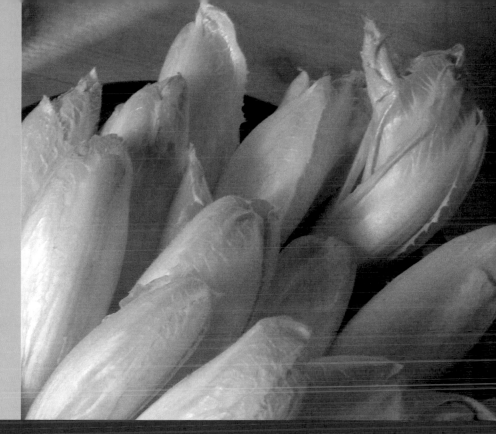

Mt. Elbert Endive

⅓ cup walnuts, coarsely chopped
2 tablespoons agave nectar, divided
½ cup balsamic vinegar
16 Belgian endive leaves
16 mandarin orange sections
⅓ cup crumbled Bleu cheese
1 tablespoon scallions, finely chopped

Per Serving:
78 Calories;
4g Fat (1g sat);
3g Protein;
9g Carbohydrate;
1g Dietary Fiber;
4mg Cholesterol;
67mg Sodium.

Combine walnuts and 1 tablespoon agave. Spray a small skillet with cooking spray and heat over medium. Add walnuts to skillet. Stir the walnuts frequently to prevent burning. As they become more fragrant and the agave appears to adhere to the walnuts (about 5 minutes), remove from heat and spread on a piece of aluminum foil until they have cooled.

While the walnuts are cooling, combine 1 tablespoon agave and balsamic vinegar in a small saucepan. Bring to a boil over high heat; lower heat, stir, and reduce to approximately 3 tablespoons (about 5 minutes) or until balsamic vinegar has more of a thick, syrupy consistency.

Arrange individual endive leaves on a serving platter. Fill each endive leaf with 1 mandarin section. Add 1 teaspoon cheese and 1 teaspoon of walnuts to each leaf. Drizzle vinegar mixture evenly over leaves; sprinkle with scallions.

Quandary Peak Quesadillas

Two words: decadent and delicious. No guilt is involved of course, since these are mere first course and the nutritionals are actually pretty awesome so enjoy!

Serves 4

1 small red onion, thinly sliced
1 tablespoon olive oil
2 whole wheat tortillas
2 ounces brie, thinly sliced
1 medium Bosc pear, cored and thinly sliced

In a medium sized skillet, heat olive oil over medium high heat. Add sliced onions. Gently stir-fry over medium-high heat until onions caramelize. Set aside. Place one tortilla in the same skillet (you may need to lightly coat is with cooking oil spray) and layer with half an ounce of sliced Brie, about 5 slices of pear, and half of the caramelized onions. Fold tortilla in half and cook over low heat, gently flipping midway through until cheese has melted. Cut each half into four slices. Serving size is 2 slices.

Per Serving:
187 Calories;
9g Fat (3g sat);
6g Protein;
23g Carbohydrate;
3g Dietary Fiber;
14mg Cholesterol;
280mg Sodium.

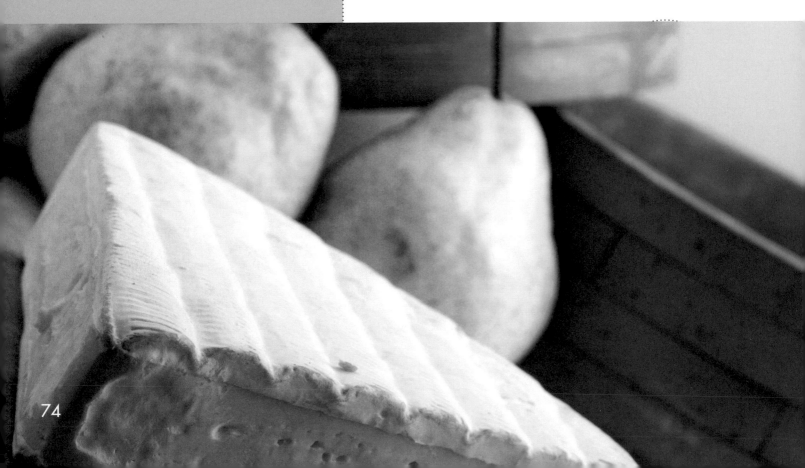

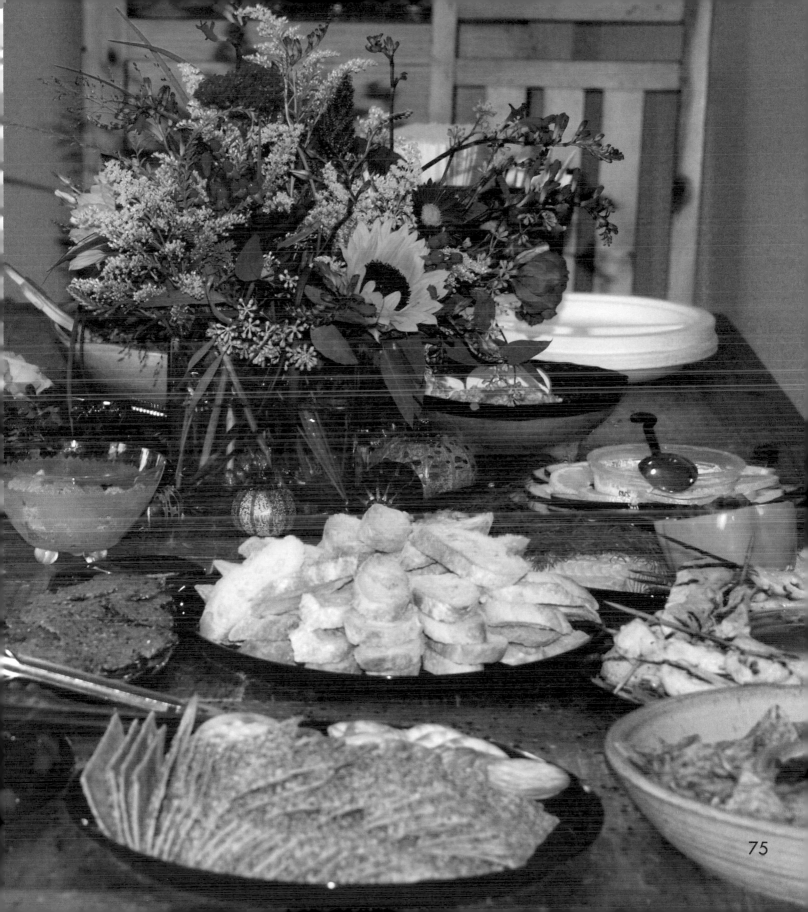

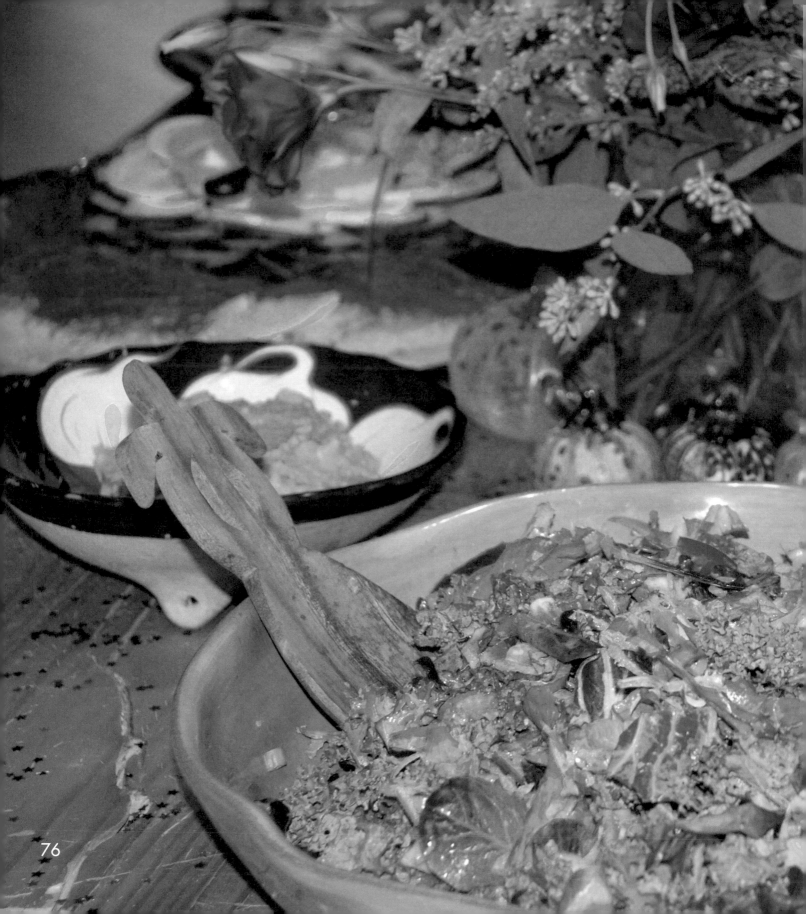

Let food be thy medicine, thy medicine shall be thy food. ~ Hippocrates

The "S" Factor:
Salads, Sandwiches,
Soups, and Sides

We could have called this section "The Lunch Factor" since many of these dishes make the perfect lunch, but truly they are all appropriate for any time of day. Combine one of the salads with one of the soups and you've got yourself an awesome meal. Many of the salad dressings are interchangeable with any of the salads. Most of the recipes are gluten-free, and keep in mind that most everything can be made gluten-free or dairy-free simply by substituting gluten-free bread, rice flour, soy milk , hemp milk, or almond milk.

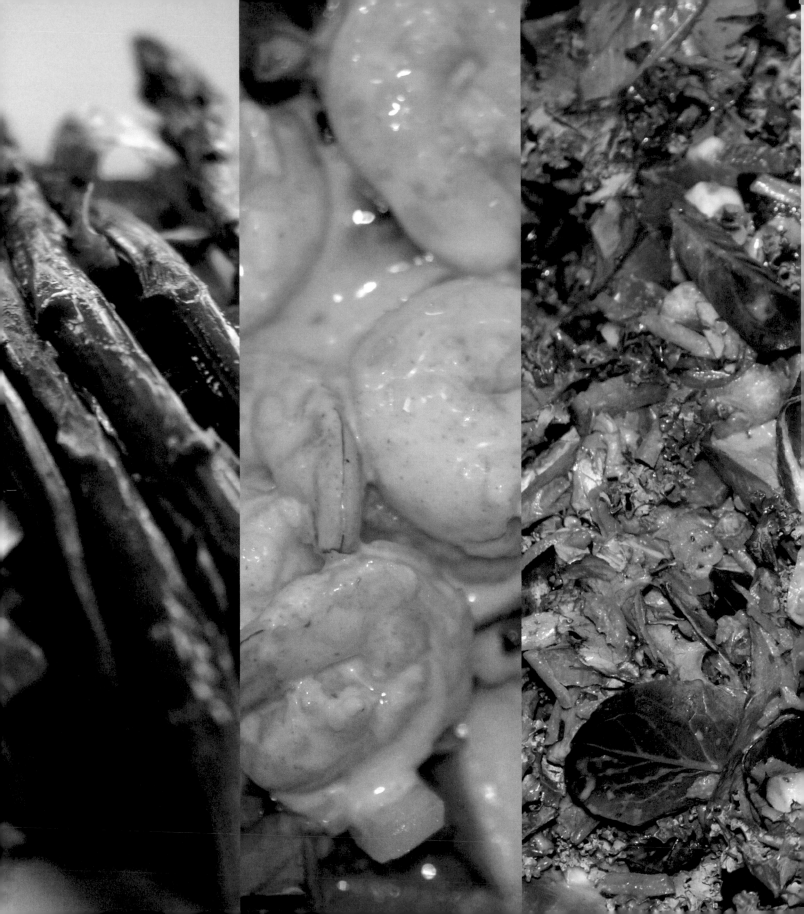

Your imagination is your preview of life's coming attractions. ~ Albert Einstein

Salads

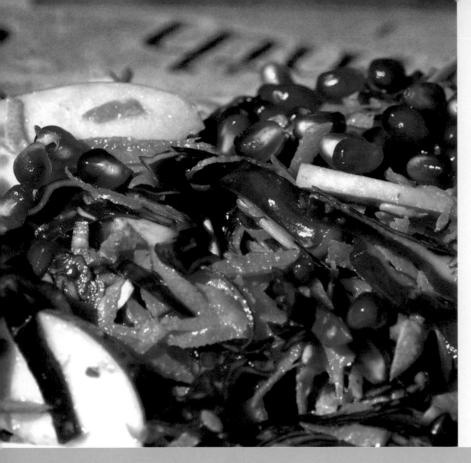

For this antioxidant-rich salad feel free to use either purple or green cabbage – both are loaded with powerful phytonutrients. The juice from pomegranate seeds has been shown effective in reducing the risk of heart disease and is being studied for its effects on type 2 diabetes, prostate cancer, lymphoma, the common cold and coronary artery disease.

Serves 4

Crunchy Munchy Slaw

Combine cabbage with carrots and apple. Transfer to a serving bowl, add sunflower seeds and mix gently. In a small bowl combine lime juice with yogurt and honey. Add to cabbage mixture and toss well to coat. Divide onto four salad plates and sprinkle top of each with one tablespoon of pomegranate seeds. Garnish with fresh cilantro or fresh mint.

4 cups cabbage, shredded
4 carrots, shredded
1 Granny Smith apple, thinly sliced or chopped
¼ cup sunflower seeds
1½ teaspoons lime juice
¼ cup nonfat yogurt
1 teaspoon honey
fresh mint or cilantro
¼ cup pomegranate, seeds

Per Serving:
139 Calories;
5g Fat (1g sat);
5g Protein;
22g Carbohydrate;
6g Dietary Fiber;
trace Cholesterol;
53mg Sodium.

Sunshine Peak Salad

This is a quick and easy salad full of terrific flavor. Plenty of health benefits to be had from the curry, yogurt, ginger, and greens!

Serves 4

¼ cup plain yogurt
¼ cup lowfat mayonnaise
1 tablespoon curry powder
1 tablespoon fresh lime juice
1 tablespoon agave nectar (or honey)
¼ teaspoon salt
1½ teaspoons fresh ginger,
   peeled and minced
1 pound cooked medium shrimp (deveined
   and shells removed)
8 cups mixed salad greens
½ cup sweet onion, sliced thin
¼ cup macadamia nuts, chopped (optional)
Divine Dressing (p. 82)
1 Asian pear (or regular pear), thinly sliced
½ honeydew melon, rind removed and
   thinly sliced

Per Serving:
169 Calories;
11g Fat (2g sat);
4g Protein;
16g Carbohydrate;
5g Dietary Fiber;
7mg Cholesterol;
109mg Sodium.

Combine first 7 ingredients (yogurt through ginger) in medium size bowl and mix well. Add shrimp and toss until coated. Refrigerate until ready to serve. Combine the salad greens, macadamia nuts and onions and toss. Add a few tablespoons of Divine Dressing and toss again. Divide salad greens mixture onto four plates. Top each plate with ¼ of the shrimp mixture. Surround the salad with sliced Asian pears and melon.

Divine Dressing

This dressing is fabulous on almost any salad. We especially like it on our kale salad. It also serves as a wonderful marinade for fish or poultry. You can see with all of the options in parentheses that there are plenty of ways to add variety to the marinade. For example, for a more Italian flavor, use red wine vinegar and garlic rather than the balsamic and ginger.

Servings – About 12

½ cup olive oil
½ cup white balsamic vinegar
2 tablespoons minced shallots
1-2 tablespoons fresh minced ginger
1-2 tablespoons fresh minced basil
1 tablespoon agave nectar (or honey)
1-2 teaspoons of fresh lemon juice (or lime juice)
1 teaspoon prepared Dijon mustard
1 teaspoon wheat-free tamari
soy sauce (or ¼ teaspoon sea salt)

Per Serving:
87 Calories;
9g Fat (1g sat);
trace Protein;
2g Carbohydrate;
trace Dietary Fiber;
0mg Cholesterol;
28mg Sodium..

Combine all ingredients in a blender and purée until desired consistency is reached. We like it pretty smooth.

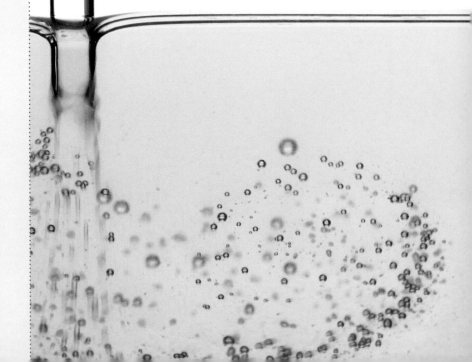

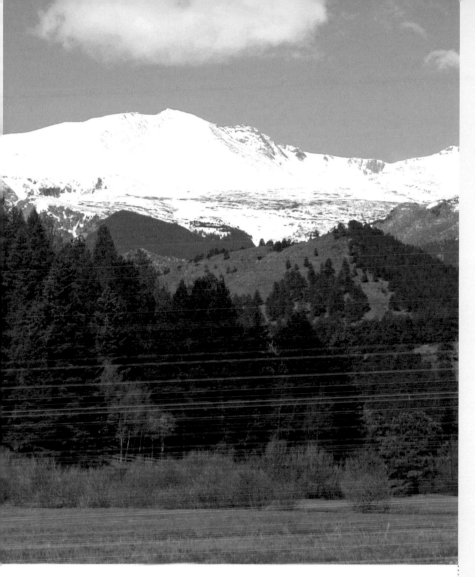

Belgian endive is a bitter type of lettuce that is a good source of fiber, vitamin A and vitamin C. Again, another healthful salad that will enliven the taste buds for sure!

Serves 4

2 tablespoons raspberry vinegar
1 tablespoon honey
1 teaspoon Dijon mustard
2 teaspoons flax seed oil
1½ tablespoons extra virgin olive oil
1 tablespoon water
¼ teaspoon sea salt
⅛ teaspoon white pepper

4 medium Belgian endive, chopped
4 cups mixed greens
1 bunch watercress
1 large pear, sliced
2 ounces chopped walnuts
1 pound cooked chicken, chopped

Whisk together raspberry vinegar through white pepper. Refrigerate until ready to use. For salad, chop endive and remove stems from watercress. Combine all the greens and toss. Gently toss in pear, walnuts and chicken. Toss in salad dressing a little at a time and serve remaining dressing on the side.

Per Serving:
385 Calories,
19g Fat (3g sat);
41g Protein;
15g Carbohydrate;
6g Dietary Fiber;
96mg Cholesterol;
240mg Sodium.

Mt. Evans Endive Salad

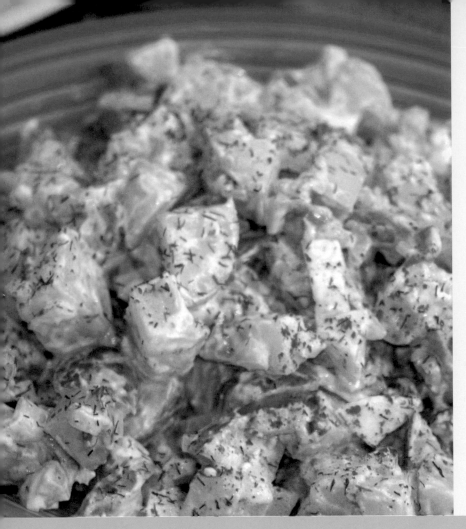

The ultimate picnic food, our version of potato salad is slightly less "dramatic" than most since we cut some of the mayonnaise and replace it with yogurt. Red potatoes actually contain a significant amount of phytonutrients and vitamins including vitamin C, folic acid, quercetin, and chemicals called kukoamines that have the potential to lower blood pressure.

Serves 6

Farmer's Market Potato Salad

Mix yogurt, mayonnaise, mustard, celery seed, salt, pepper and dill in large bowl. Add remaining ingredients; toss until vegetables are evenly coated. Cover and refrigerate at least 3 hours.

Per Serving:
171 Calories;
7g Fat (1g sat);
5g Protein;
22g Carbohydrate;
2g Dietary Fiber;
71mg Cholesterol;
500mg Sodium.

½ cup nonfat mayonnaise
¼ cup plain nonfat Greek-style yogurt
2 teaspoons Dijon mustard
½ teaspoon celery seed
½ teaspoon salt
¼ teaspoon pepper
1 teaspoon dill
3 cups red potatoes, cooked and diced
½ cup celery, diced (about 1 or 2 ribs)
½ cup kalamata (or green) olives, pitted and chopped
½ cup Vidalia onion, chopped
2 hard-cooked eggs, chopped

84

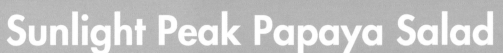

Sunlight Peak Papaya Salad

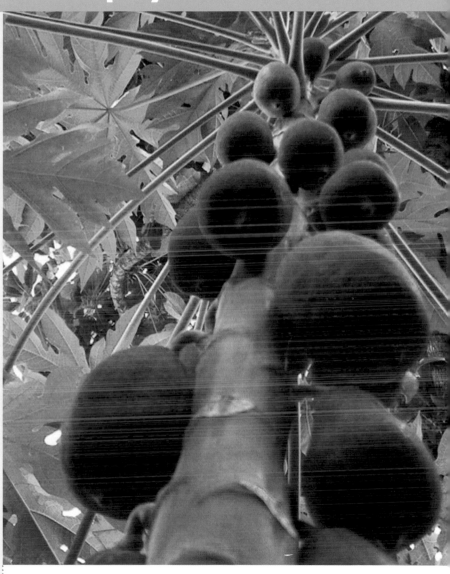

Admittedly this salad takes some time prepare, but it is certainly worth the effort. Green papaya contains an enzyme called papain, which helps with protein digestion. All of the herbs in this salad have amazing anti-inflammatory properties – you'll feel vibrant after eating it!

Serves 4

1 cup green papaya, grated
2 cups ripe papaya, diced
2 avocados, cubed
1 cup carrot, shredded
2 tablespoons grated lime zest
1 tablespoon lemon grass, finely minced
½ cup red bell pepper, diced
¼ cup red onion, chopped
¼ cup shallot, chopped
½ cup cucumber, sliced
½ cup fresh cilantro, chopped
1 cup fresh mint, chopped
½ cup fresh basil, chopped
1 tablespoon garlic, minced
½ tablespoon ginger, minced
1 tablespoon curry powder
1 tablespoon tamari soy sauce
¼ cup fresh squeezed lime juice
¼ cup fresh squeezed orange juice
16 ounces firm tofu, cubed (*you can
    substitute small cooked shrimp for the tofu)
Lime wedges for garnish

Combine all of the ingredients in a large bowl and toss together lightly. Serve with lime wedges.

Per Serving:
230 Calories;
14g Fat (2g sat);
10g Protein;
22g Carbohydrate;
6g Dietary Fiber;
0mg Cholesterol;
197mg Sodium.

85

Whole-Hearted Salad

This is definitely a summery salad. It has always been a favorite at our post-tennis socials. Of course we can't say enough about the benefits of blueberries – loaded with phytochemicals that may prevent free-radical damage linked to heart disease and cancer. Get them at the peak of the season, which is generally May through July in North America.

Serves 4

16 ounces cooked chicken breast
   halves, chopped, shredded or cubed
1 small red onion, cut in ¼-inch strips
8 cups mixed greens, can mix in spinach
¼ cup chopped pecans
½ cup blueberries
⅓ cup balsamic vinegar, or red wine vinegar
¼ cup honey
2 teaspoons Dijon mustard
1 clove garlic, minced
1 teaspoon Italian seasoning
¼ teaspoon salt and pepper
1 tablespoon olive oil

Per Serving:
386 Calories;
16g Fat (3g sat);
32g Protein;
32g Carbohydrate;
6g Dietary Fiber;
77mg Cholesterol;
217mg Sodium.

In a large salad bowl, toss together chicken through blueberries. In a blender or mason jar, blend or shake together balsamic vinegar through olive oil. Drizzle dressing over salad and toss again to coat. Divide salad onto four salad plates or bowls and enjoy.

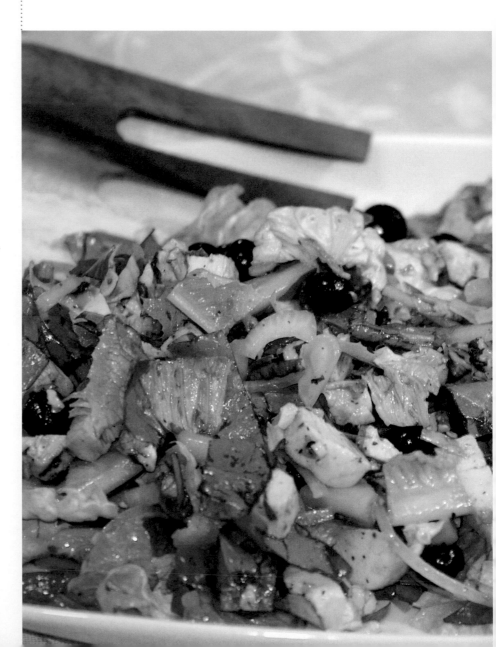

86

Mediterranean Chopped Veggie Salad

We make many versions of this scrumptious summertime salad. Start by thoroughly washing all the vegetables, removing seeds and stems from the peppers, and drying so that there isn't a lot of water left on the surface. To roast the vegetables we usually cut the peppers into quarters and slice the zucchini into about 4 or 5 long slices, same with the eggplant. We cut the onion into quarters because we find they are easier to grill or roast this way. We usually roast the vegetables in the oven on a broiling pan or grill them. We either spray them lightly with olive oil spray or use a pastry brush to lightly coat them in olive oil. We also sprinkle them lightly with salt and pepper.

After grilling all of the vegetables, we wait for them to cool. Then we proceed to chop away, adding them all to a large mixing bowl. After all the veggies are cooled and chopped, we add the goat cheese, olives, and artichoke hearts and toss until well combined. We drizzle about a tablespoon of olive oil and red wine vinegar (or balsamic) over the salad and toss it together. We'll taste it before deciding whether or not to add more salt. It usually doesn't need it because the feta adds quite a bit of saltiness, as do the olives.

Serving size is about one cup.

This amazing salad was developed after we ended up with a lot of leftover roasted vegetables following a party. We diced and chopped, added a little feta, a few artichoke hearts and some olives and a new favorite was born. Loaded with heart-healthy phytonutrients, vitamins, and minerals, we trust you'll love it like we do.

Serves 4

2 red peppers, roasted and chopped - about ½ cup
2 yellow bell peppers, roasted and chopped
1 zucchini, sliced lengthwise, then roasted and chopped
½ cup eggplant, sliced lengthwise, then roasted and chopped
1 small red onion, cut into quarters and roasted
2 large Portobello mushroom caps, roasted and chopped
¼ cup pitted black olives, chopped
½ cup marinated artichoke hearts, chopped
2 tablespoons crumbled feta cheese
1 tablespoon olive oil
1 tablespoon red wine vinegar
salt and pepper

Per Serving:
151 Calories;
7g Fat (1g sat);
5g Protein;
19g Carbohydrate;
5g Dietary Fiber;
4mg Cholesterol;
229mg Sodium.

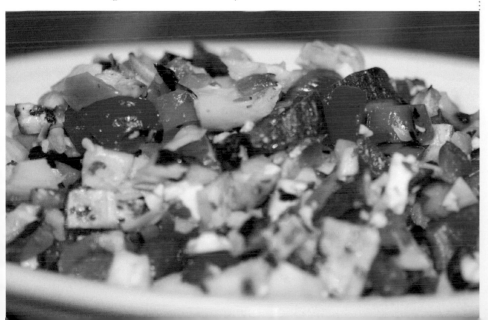

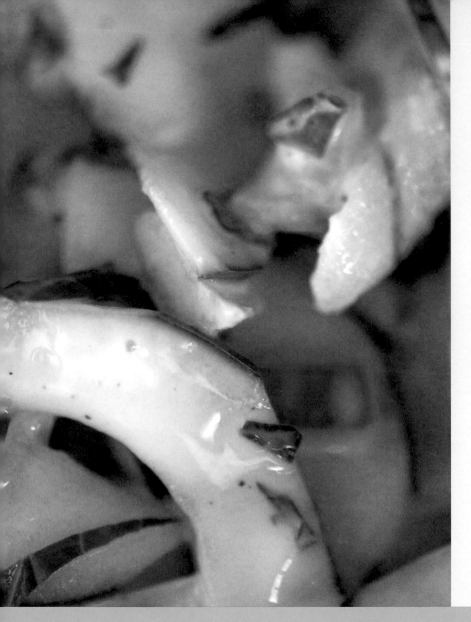

Cucumbers contain silica, which is a mineral essential for connective tissue, bone, hair, skin, and nails. They also contain vitamin C, fiber, potassium, and magnesium. This is a wonderfully cooling salad – for a dairy-free version you can go without the yogurt.

Serves 4

Per Serving:
56 Calories;
2g Fat (1g sat);
3g Protein;
7g Carbohydrate;
1g Dietary Fiber;
8mg Cholesterol;
298mg Sodium

Minted Cucumber Salad

Cut ends off of cucumbers and slice lengthwise. Remove seeds and thinly slice cucumber in half moon shape. Combine all ingredients together and enjoy!

2 small cucumbers
¼ cup red onion, chopped
2 tablespoons rice vinegar
1 teaspoon sugar
½ teaspoon salt
½ teaspoon pepper
1 cup plain yogurt
3 tablespoons fresh mint, chopped

For the pasta lovers, we had to include this salad. We usually use gluten-free penne pasta, which holds up well to the tossing. We boosted the antioxidant and fiber content by adding all of the fabulous ingredients you see here. This is a perfect potluck or picnic dish. Experiment with various fresh herbs like fresh mint, basil, thyme or rosemary. Sundried tomatoes or artichoke hearts also make a nice addition.

Serves 10

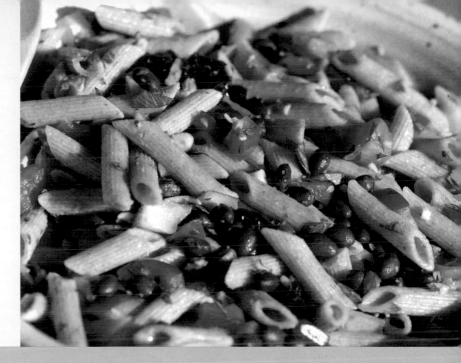

Pike's Peak Pasta Salad

1 pound penne pasta
½ teaspoon salt, optional
2 tablespoons fresh lime juice (about ½ lime)
1 tablespoon olive oil
½ cup toasted almonds, chopped
½ cup dried cranberries
½ cup diced red onion
1 medium red bell pepper, seeded and diced
1 medium tomato, diced
15 ounces black beans, (1 can rinsed and drained)
2 tablespoons fresh parsley
1 tablespoon fresh cilantro
¼ teaspoon seasoned salt (optional)
¼ teaspoon black pepper

Per Serving:
384 Calories;
7g Fat (1g sat);
17g Protein;
64g Carbohydrate;
9g Dietary Fiber;
0mg Cholesterol;
149mg Sodium.

Bring 4 quarts of water with ½ teaspoon of salt to a rapid boil. Add pasta and cook until done al dente (see package for approximate cooking times). When pasta is done cooking rinse with cool water and drain.

Add cooked pasta to large bowl and toss with a tablespoon of olive oil. Add fresh lime juice and toss to coat. Add remaining ingredients (almonds through salt and pepper). Toss well to combine. Refrigerate until ready to serve.

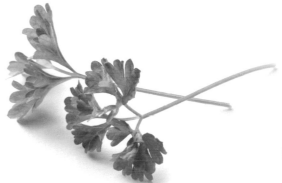

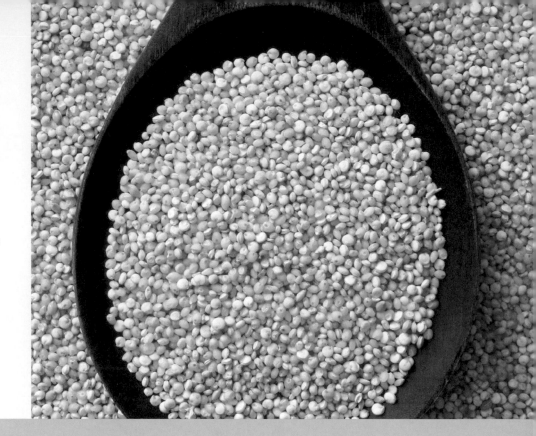

Black currants are loaded with antioxidants, vitamins, minerals and even essential fatty acids (gamma-linoleic acid). The anthocyanins in currants may help reduce inflammation in the body. We like to add them to salads and baked goods whenever we can.

Serves 4

Quinoa, Chicken and Currant Salad

1 cup quinoa, well rinsed and drained
2 cups low sodium chicken broth
2 cups cooked chicken breast
¼ cup dried currants
¼ cup green onion, finely chopped
1 tablespoon olive oil
1 tablespoon fresh lemon juice
salt and pepper, to taste

Per Serving:
363 Calories;
9g Fat (2g sat);
33g Protein;
38g Carbohydrate;
3g Dietary Fiber;
60mg Cholesterol;
324mg Sodium.

Rinse quinoa in a bowl or fine strainer until water runs clear (you may need several changes of water).

Add quinoa and chicken broth to medium-sized stockpot and bring to a boil. Lower heat to simmer and cover. Quinoa is quick cooking and should only take around 15 minutes to cook. While quinoa is cooking, shred the cooked chicken either by hand or with forks.

When quinoa is ready (fluffy), add remaining ingredients to the pot and stir to combine. Allow the salad to "rest" for a few minutes to allow the flavors to begin to set. You can serve this dish warm or cold. This also makes a great snack anytime of day.

Rainbow Salad

Wash and dry romaine lettuce leaves. You'll want to use the freshest of the leaves and chop into thin ribbons until you have about 6 cups. Add the rest of the salad ingredients (cabbage though avocado) and toss to combine.

We often toss this with Divine Dressing (p. 82) or Almond Butter Dressing (p. 235) and add grilled chicken or salmon.

Per Serving:
79 Calories;
6g Fat (1g sat);
3g Protein;
7g Carbohydrate;
3g Dietary Fiber;
0mg Cholesterol;
17mg Sodium.

Serves 4

1 head romaine lettuce, washed and chopped
   into thin ribbons
1 cup shredded cabbage
½ cup shredded carrots
¼ cup green onions, chopped
1 medium red bell pepper, seeded and chopped
¼ cup vinaigrette

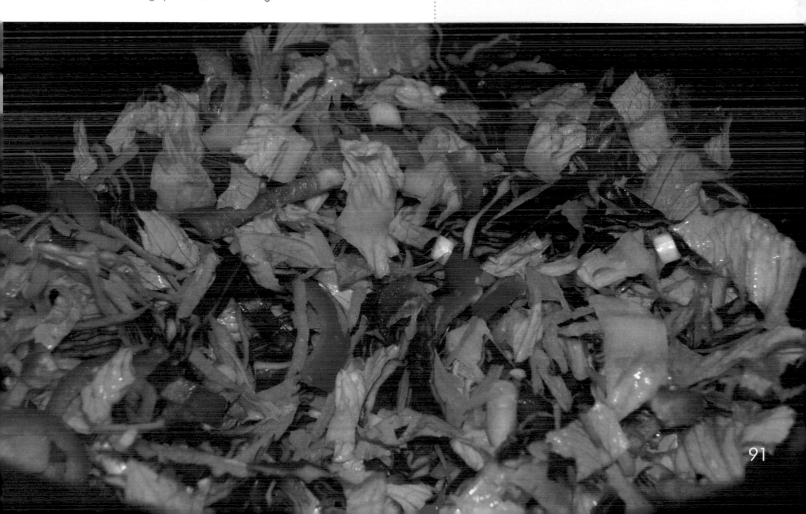

91

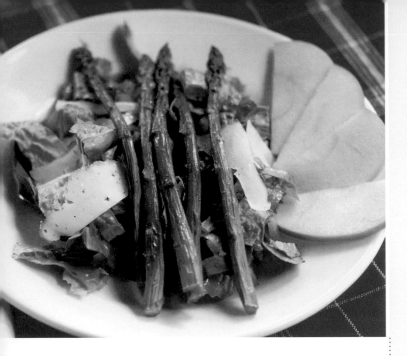

Whisk together olive oil, raspberry vinegar, and honey or shake together in mason jar with tight fitting lid.

Preheat oven to 400°F. Rinse asparagus and remove tough ends. Drizzle with 1 tablespoon olive oil and toss to coat. Sprinkle lightly with sea salt and pepper. Line a baking sheet with parchment and set the asparagus on the parchment in a single layer. Roast for about 8 minutes and then turn them over and roast an additional 8 minutes on the other side. Allow to cool at least 5 minutes.

Rinse and dry the lettuce and place in a large bowl. Season with a small amount of dressing – enough to lightly coat the lettuce. Toss in the cheese and the apple slices or you may choose to garnish each plate with these items. Place a good helping of salad on each plate and top with about 5 asparagus spears.

Serve with additional dressing on the side.

Asparagus gets its name from the Greek word (asparagus) for sprout or shoot. Asparagus is a wonderful food, high in fiber, vitamin C, folate, iron, and B vitamins. When picking out Asparagus (the green variety), look for stalks that are firm, not slimy, and with deep green or purplish tips.

You'll want to eat the asparagus right away – the fresher the better. Keep fresh asparagus cold to preserve the natural sweetness and vitamin C. Even just kept at room temperature, the asparagus can lose half it's vitamin C in 2 days.

If you're wondering why your urine smells funny after you eat asparagus, don't worry, you're not alone. Roughly 40% of us have an enzyme that causes us to excrete a sulfur compound from asparagus that has a distinct sulfurous odor.

Serves 4

25 asparagus spears
1 tablespoon olive oil
1 dash sea salt
1 dash black pepper
6 cups romaine lettuce, shredded
1 medium Granny Smith apple, quartered and sliced
2 ounces Manchego-style sheep's milk cheese shredded or cut into ribbons with a veggie peeler (or use crumbled goat cheese)
2 tablespoons olive oil
¼ cup raspberry vinegar
1 tablespoon honey

Per Serving
(Based on the use of goat cheese):
222 Calories; 16g Fat (5g sat);
8g Protein;16g Carbohydrate;
4g Dietary Fiber;
15mg Cholesterol;
118mg Sodium.

Roasted Asparagus Salad

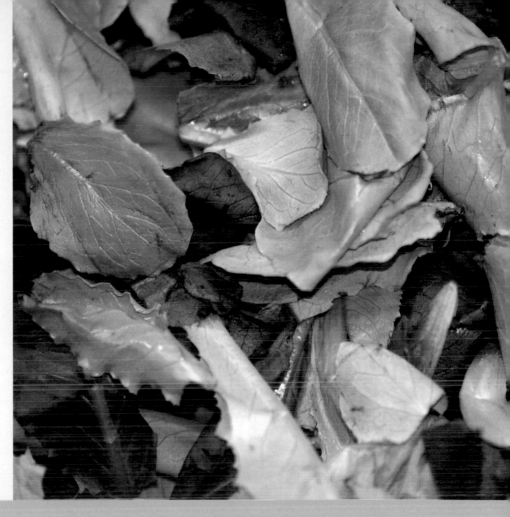

Alas, our version of the basic, and delightful salad.

Serves 5

Salad Greens with Lemon Basil Vinaigrette

10 cups greens
½ cup carrot, grated
2 tomatoes, chopped
½ cup zucchini, chopped
½ cup red onion, chopped

Vinaigrette
¼ cup fresh basil, chopped
1 tablespoon Dijon mustard
½ teaspoon sea salt
½ teaspoon lemon pepper
½ cup olive oil
¼ cup balsamic vinegar
1 tablespoon fresh lemon juice

In a large bowl, toss greens, carrot, tomatoes, zucchini, and red onion.

Prepare Lemon Basil Vinaigrette by shaking all ingredients together in a tightly covered jar or blending in a blender or mini processor. Shake again before pouring over salad.

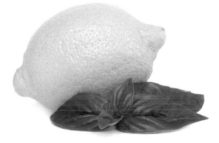

93

We like to rotate our proteins and tofu or tempeh is often included in the rotation. Regular or extra firm tofu works best in salad dishes. You can find pre-marinated/baked tofu already packaged. This makes for an easy solution to quick salads and sandwiches and solves the dilemma of finding time to marinate. If you only have access to plain tofu then a quick marinade in tamari followed by a light stir-fry should also do the trick. This recipe is loaded with phytonutrients from the broccoli sprouts to the tomatoes. The dressing is reminiscent of a Thai peanut sauce — made with almonds, of course.

Serves 6

For the dressing, combine all the ingredients in a blender and blend until smooth and creamy.

Add the snap beans, carrot, broccoli sprouts, scallions, tomato, and mixed greens to a large salad bowl. Top with half the almond butter dressing and toss. Divide the greens mixture among 6 salad plates. Top each salad with ½ cup tofu. Garnish with chopped almonds, mint, and cilantro. Serve with additional dressing.

Savory Tofu Salad with Almond Butter Dressing

Per Serving
(w/o dressing):
136 Calories;
6g fat (1g sat); 13g Protein;
12g Carbohydrate;
4g Dietary Fiber;
0mg Cholesterol;
37mg Sodium.

*3 cups marinated baked savory tofu, cubed
(you can find this in the refrigerated section of most
   natural food stores and selected groceries)
1 cup snap beans, lightly steamed and cooled
1 carrot, peeled and julienned
1 cup broccoli sprouts
½ cup scallions, chopped
1 cup plum tomato, diced
6 cups mixed greens*

*Dressing:
½ cup tofu
3 tablespoons almond butter
2 tablespoons wheat-free tamari soy sauce
4 tablespoons rice vinegar
2 tablespoons agave syrup
1½ tablespoons fresh ginger, peeled and chopped
4 tablespoons light coconut milk
1 scallion, finely chopped*

*Garnish:
6 tablespoons almonds, chopped
6 teaspoons fresh mint, chopped
6 teaspoons fresh cilantro, chopped*

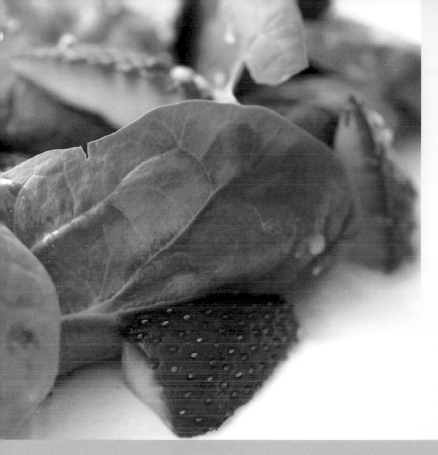

This type of salad appears on many summer menus. We love the combination of the fresh strawberries with the chevre. If you are not a fan of goat cheese, you can substitute feta or leave out the cheese altogether. We always choose organic strawberries since non-organic strawberries always top the list of the "dirty dozen" for high pesticide residues (even after washing).

Serves 4

Per Serving:
333 Calories;
27g Fat (5g sat);
15g Protein;
14g Carbohydrate;
5g Dietary Fiber;
15mg Cholesterol;
125mg Sodium.

Spinach Strawberry Salad with Chevre

Prepare Agave-Mustard Dressing by shaking all ingredients together in a tightly covered jar or blending in a blender or mini processor. Shake again before pouring over salad.

Rinse the strawberries with cool water, and pat dry. Remove the leaves, and cut the berries lengthwise into slices.

Rinse the spinach well and spin or pat dry. Do the same with the mixed greens. Add both to a large salad bowl. Add the strawberries, kiwis and walnuts to the bowl of greens, pour the dressing over the ingredients, and toss. Add in crumbled chevre cheese and toss again gently.

Agave-Mustard Dressing:
1 tablespoon olive oil
1 tablespoon flax seed oil
2 tablespoons agave syrup (or honey)
1 tablespoon orange juice
1 tablespoon lime juice
1 tablespoon rice wine vinegar
2 teaspoons Dijon mustard

1 cup organic strawberries, chopped
½ cup kiwi fruit, peeled and chopped
6 cups fresh spinach, well rinsed and drained
2 cups mixed greens, well rinsed and drained
1 cup walnuts, chopped
½ cup crumbled chevre (from a plain log or feta)

A simple twist on your basic tuna salad. You can also substitute pre-cooked chicken or salmon in this recipe. It's a great balance of whole grains and quality protein.

Serves 6

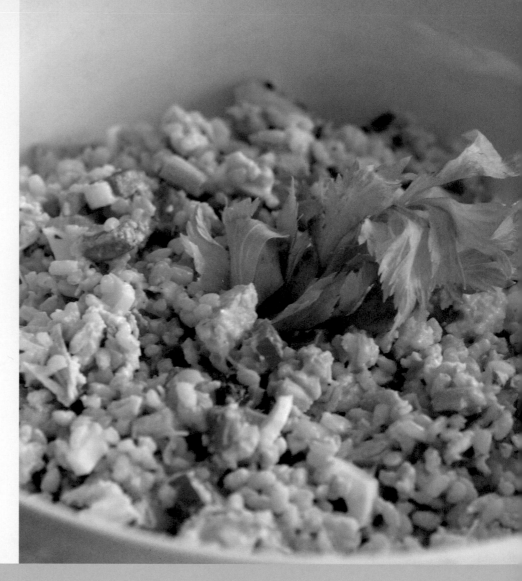

Per Serving:
274Calories;
8g Fat (2g sat);
14g Protein;
35g Carbohydrate;
3g Dietary Fiber;
69mg Cholesterol;
321mg Sodium.

Shine Your Light Rice Salad

2 ½ cups brown rice, cooked
1 12-ounce can tuna, packed in water
1 egg, hard-boiled and crumbled
2 celery stalks, chopped
2 green onions, chopped
½ cup light mayonnaise
1 tablespoon fresh lemon juice
½ teaspoon Dijon mustard
salt and pepper, as desired

Combine rice through green onions and toss until mixed. Whisk together mayonnaise, lemon juice, and mustard, and toss with tuna and rice salad. Add salt and pepper to taste.

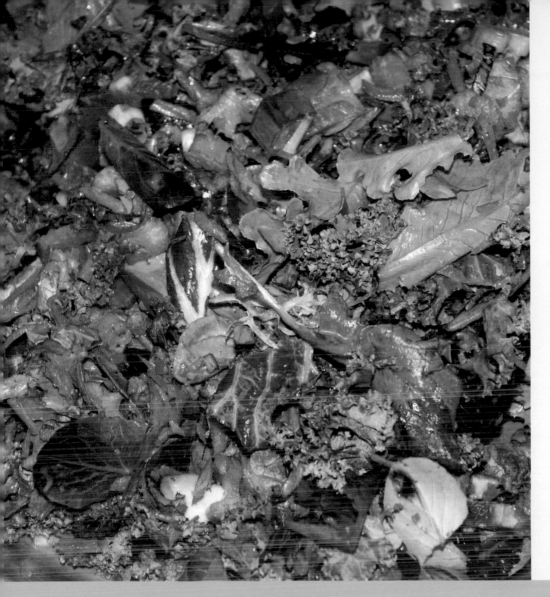

Our kale salad is always a hit at potlucks and usually the healthiest dish on the table. When you tell friends and family about the many health benefits of kale – including cutting our risk for developing many cancers, decreasing risk for cataracts, supporting the immune system, protecting against rheumatoid arthritis, benefitting mental health, protecting the heart and providing a great source of calcium – they'll appreciate eating it that much more!

Serves 6

Per Serving:
88 Calories;
5g Fat (1g sat);
3g Protein;
10g Carbohydrate;
3g Dietary Fiber;
0mg Cholesterol;
w30mg Sodium.

Kale Salad

Rinse and spin or towel-dry the kale. Remove leaves from the stem. Roughly chop the kale into small pieces and place them in a large bowl. Make sure mixed greens are also well washed and dried and add them to the kale. Add the remaining ingredients and toss to combine. We recommend serving this salad with Divine Dressing (p. 82).

3 cups kale
3 cups mixed greens
½ cup shredded carrots
½ cup red bell pepper, chopped
½ cup scallions, chopped
1 medium avocado, chopped

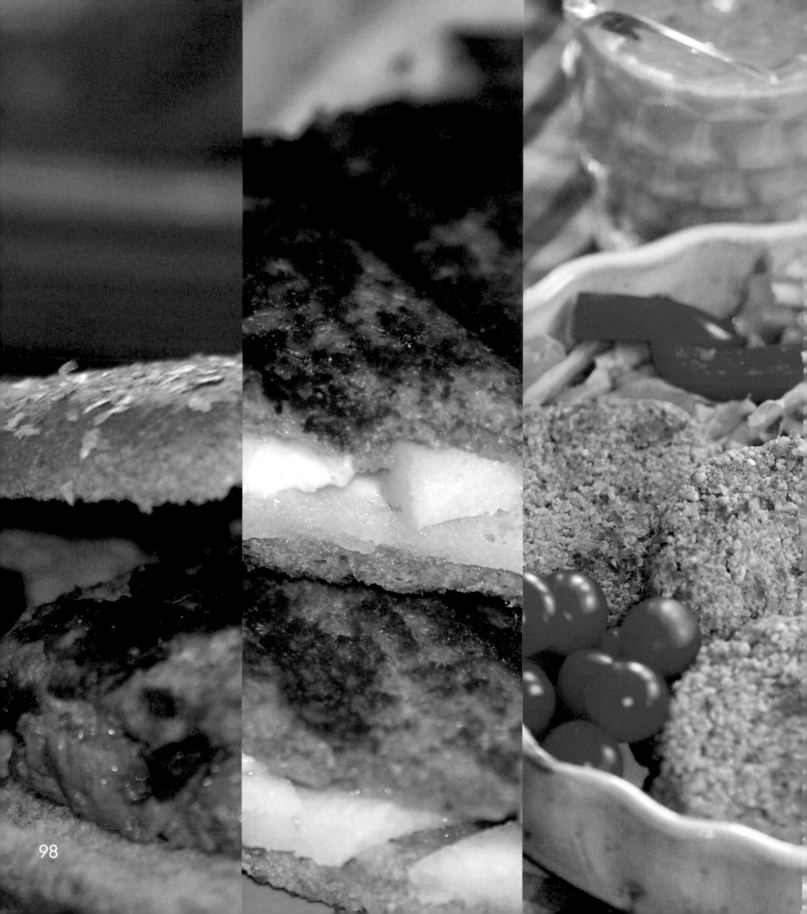

Too few people understand a really good sandwich. ~James Beard

Sandwiches

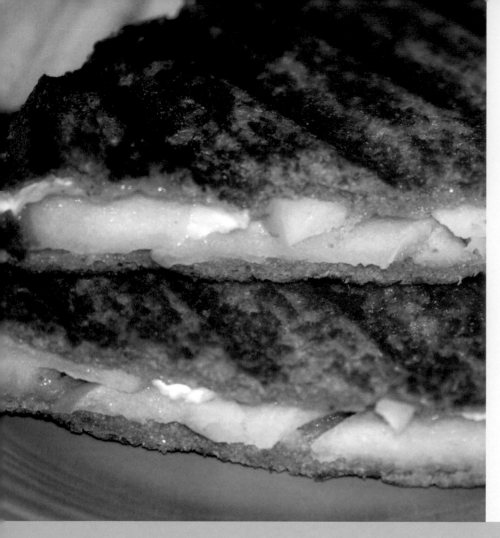

This sandwich cooks up really quickly and can be a fun alternative to your typical grilled sandwich. As an alternative, you can cut it into small pieces and serve as an appetizer during the holidays.

Serves 1

Apple-Brie Sandwich

Lightly coat the outside of two pieces of whole grain bread with olive oil spray or a very thin layer of butter.

If you like you may spread the inside of one slice with mustard. Layer the apple slices and brie on one slice of bread, then top with the other.

Heat a nonstick skillet over medium-high. Place the prepared sandwich on the skillet and grill over medium for about 3 minutes each side - or until Brie just starts to melt.

½ *medium Granny Smith apple, sliced*
1 *ounce Brie*
2 *whole wheat bread slices*
mustard, optional

Per Serving:
263 Calories; 10g Fat
(5g sat); 12g Protein;
34g Carbohydrate;
5g Dietary Fiber;
28mg Cholesterol;
475mg Sodium.

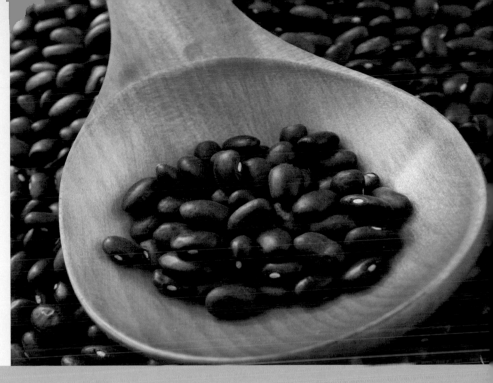

A nice alternative to beef burgers and loaded with antioxidants, fiber, and immune-boosting phytochemicals.

Makes 4 burgers

Shadow Mountain Burgers

1 can (15 ounces) cooked black beans
1 tablespoon horseradish mustard
2 tablespoons tomato paste
1 tablespoon flour
1 teaspoon ground cumin
1 tablespoon olive oil
1 garlic clove, minced
¼ cup minced onion
¼ cup shiitake mushrooms, chopped
cooking spray
2 tablespoons almonds
1 piece whole wheat bread, toasted

Per Serving:
281 Calories;
7g Fat (1g sat);
13g Protein;
45g Carbohydrate;
13g Dietary Fiber;
0mg Cholesterol;
163mg Sodium.

Drain black beans of any liquid and place in a medium size bowl. Mash with a fork and add mustard, tomato paste, flour and cumin.

Meanwhile, add 1 tablespoon olive oil to a medium hot skillet. Add onion, garlic and mushrooms and sauté about 5 minutes or until mushrooms are tender. Add to black bean mixture and stir until well mixed. Form the mixture into 4 burgers.

In a toaster or warm oven, toast whole wheat bread until it dries out but isn't burnt. Tear bread into pieces and process with almonds in a food processor or coffee grinder until well ground. Dip each black bean patty into the bread/almond mixture on each side. Grill each black bean patty on a skillet coated with cooking spray heated on medium high. Cook each side about 3 to 4 minutes or until desired doneness. Serve on salad greens, on a whole wheat bun or English muffin.

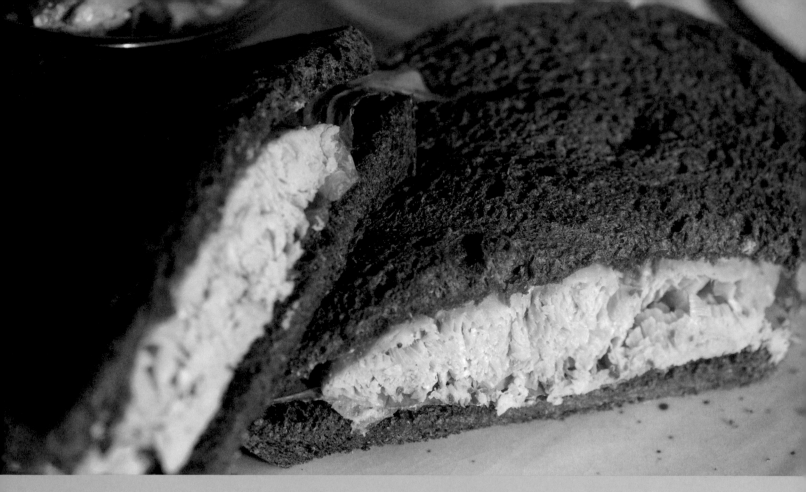

River Runner Salmon Sandwich

Serves 4

1 pound salmon fillet
¼ cup Dijon mustard
2 tablespoons honey
1 teaspoon dried oregano
⅛ teaspoon ground red pepper
¼ teaspoon garlic powder
1 teaspoon water
4 large romaine lettuce leaves
8 slices pumpernickel bread
2 teaspoons lowfat mayonnaise
2 tablespoons scallions, chopped

Mix mustard, honey, oregano, garlic powder, red pepper and water; brush on salmon. Heat coals or gas grill. Cover and grill salmon about 15 minutes, brushing with mustard mixture and turning once until fish flakes easily with a fork. Discard any remaining mustard mixture.

After salmon is cooked to your liking, remove skin and divide into 4 pieces.

Lightly toast or grill each bread slice and serve salmon on top of lettuce. You may opt to add chopped scallions and ½ teaspoon mayonnaise to your sandwich.

Per Serving:
346 Calories;
7g Fat (1g sat);
29g Protein;
41g Carbohydrate;
5g Dietary Fiber;
60mg Cholesterol;
707mg Sodium.

Ginger Chicken Spring Rolls

Marinate chicken in ginger marinade for a few hours.

Meanwhile prepare dipping sauce by combining first 5 ingredients in a medium saucepan and bring to a boil while stirring. Remove from heat and whisk in peanut butter. When cool, add cilantro and mint.

When ready to prepare chicken, either grill over medium high or bake at 350°F for about 20 minutes. When chicken has cooled, either chop finely with knife or shred in food processor.

Pour boiling or very hot tap water into a large shallow bowl. Add rice paper one at a time for about 15 seconds until soft. Gently remove rice paper and layer ½ leaf of lettuce plus 1½ tablespoons chicken and a few mint and cilantro springs. Roll in sides then roll up like a burrito. Serve with dipping sauce.

Per Serving:
235 Calories;
5g Fat (1g sat)
18g Protein;
30g Carbohydrate;
1g Dietary Fiber;
33mg Cholesterol;
583mg Sodium.

These spring rolls make a delightful lunch entree or a substantial appetizer. (see also Shrimp Spring Rolls p. 70)

Serves 4

½ cup Prepared ginger marinade (We use Annie's Organic Ginger Marinade)
1 pound boneless skinless chicken breast
1 head of butter lettuce
Rice paper
Fresh mint and cilantro for garnish

Dipping Sauce:
¼ cup balsamic vinegar
2 tablespoons sugar
2 tablespoons brown sugar
½ teaspoon crushed red pepper
2 tablespoons tamari soy sauce
2 tablespoons peanut butter
½ cup fresh chopped cilantro
2 tablespoons fresh chopped mint

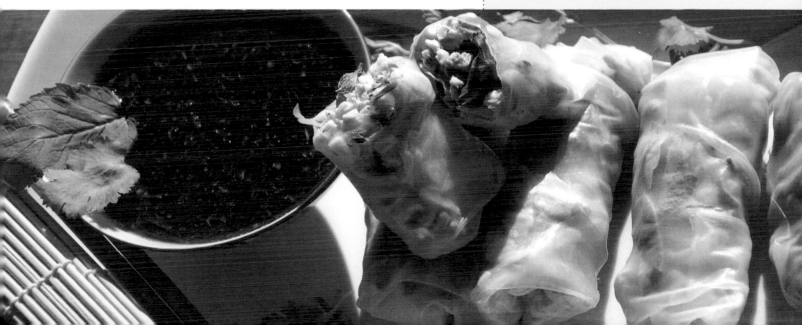

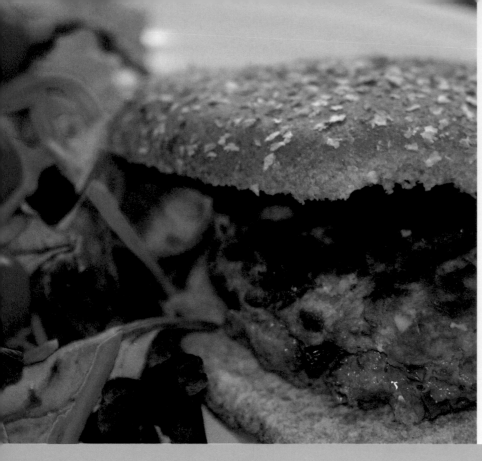

We usually make these burgers with ground turkey. The surprising filling is delicious and as a result you won't need a lot of condiments with these burgers.

Serves 4

Mark's Burger

Combine ground beef or turkey with breadcrumbs, lemon juice and peel, thyme, salt and pepper and chopped sun dried tomatoes. Mix well and divide mixture into 4 portions. Divide each portion in half and form small round patties. (Do this with each of the four portions). Place a tablespoon of goat cheese in the center of one patty and place a second patty on top. Press edges of patty together to form a seal - so that your two patties become one patty with the goat cheese in the middle.

Heat grill to medium-high. Grill burgers until cooked through - about five minutes each side (or a little less if using ground turkey).

Serve burgers with condiments of choice or serve over mixed greens.

1 pound ground lean beef or turkey
4 tablespoons bread crumbs
1 tablespoon lemon juice
1 teaspoon lemon peel
1 teaspoon dried thyme
½ teaspoon sea salt
¼ teaspoon ground black pepper
½ cup sun-dried tomatoes, chopped
4 tablespoons goat cheese

Per Serving:
363 Calories;
6g Fat (10g sat);
15g Protein;
9g Carbohydrate;
1g Dietary Fiber;
38mg Cholesterol;
482mg Sodium.

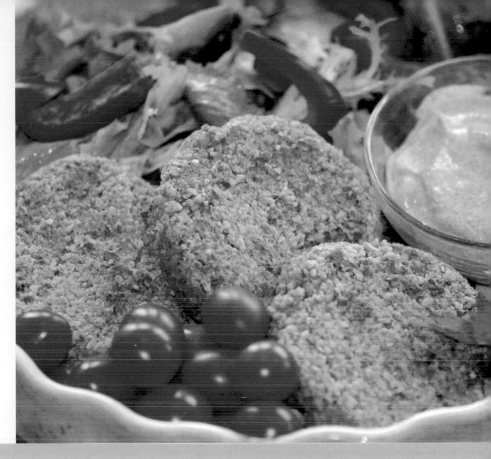

Sunflower seeds are laden with vitamin E, a fat-soluble antioxidant vitamin that our bodies need. Sunflower seeds also contain magnesium (think heart, bone, and nerve health and energy production) and vitamin B1 (thiamine) (also energy and nerves).

Serves 6

Sunflower Burgers

2 cups sunflower seeds
1 cup cooked brown rice
½ cup grated carrots
1 teaspoon parsley
1 teaspoon salt
1 teaspoon sage
1 teaspoon black pepper

Per Serving:
394 Calories;
25g Fat (3g sat);
13g Protein;
34g Carbohydrate;
6g Dietary Fiber;
0mg Cholesterol;
362mg Sodium.

Add all ingredients to food processor and process until chunky paste like consistency develops. Divide mixture into 4 to 6 balls and form into patties. Brown patties on both sides in a lightly oiled or nonstick skillet. You may also choose to cook the patties in a 350°F oven for about 20 minutes.

Other options include adding about 2 eggs to the mixture, topping with cheese or adding ½ cup grated cheese to the mixture.

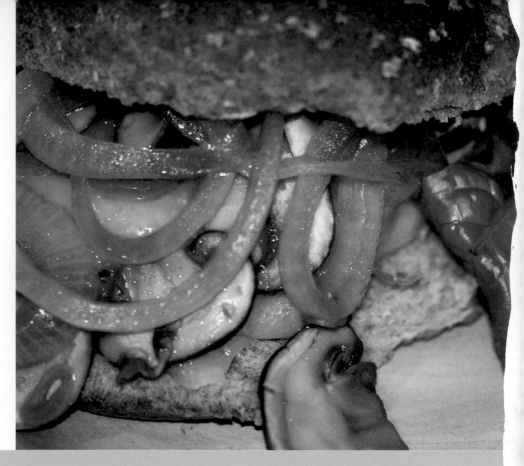

We tend to use a combination of turkey breast and turkey thigh when we make burgers. They stick together a little better and we like the richness of flavor that comes from the thigh meat.

Serves 4

Matterhorn Burger

1 cup sliced fresh shiitake
  mushrooms, rinsed and dried
1 tablespoon olive oil
1 cup yellow onion, thinly sliced
1 pound ground turkey
1 medium egg
2 tablespoons oats
2 tablespoons ketchup
½ teaspoon garlic powder
½ teaspoon black pepper
1 teaspoon oregano
4 slices Swiss cheese

4 whole grain hamburger buns
2 teaspoons brown mustard (optional)

Combine mushrooms and onions with olive oil in nonstick skillet or wok. Stir-fry until onions begin to become translucent and mushrooms are tender and golden.

Combine turkey through oregano, mixing well and divide mixture into 4 equal portions. Grill over medium high heat or pan sear on a nonstick skillet lightly coated with cooking oil until cooked. After flipping, top with one slice of Swiss cheese.

Serve burger on whole grain hamburger bun spread with brown mustard and topped with onion and mushroom mixture.

Per Serving:
449 Calories;
19g Fat (6g sat);
35g Protein;
34g Carbohydrate;
4g Dietary Fiber;
139mg Cholesterol;
396mg Sodium.

Tempeh is a fermented food made from whole soybeans. It has a higher protein, fiber, and vitamin content compared to tofu and a much firmer texture. We also find that tempeh is more digestible than tofu — a result of the fermentation process.

Serves 4

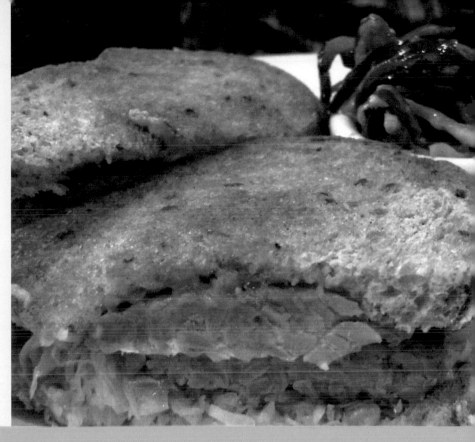

Tempeh Reuben

8 ounces Simply Tempeh (p. 190)
8 slices whole grain or rye bread
4 – 8 slices Swiss cheese (two slices on each sandwich for cheese lovers)
½ cup sauerkraut, warmed (microwave or stovetop)
4 teaspoons mustard
olive oil cooking spray

Per Serving:
478 Calories;
16g Fat (7 sat);
29g Protein;
60g Carbohydrate;
8g Dietary Fiber;
26mg Cholesterol;
625mg Sodium.

We like to make this sandwich on our George Foreman Gill or panini press, but it is almost as easily made in a skillet. Heat your press or skillet over medium heat. Lightly coat one side of each piece of bread with cooking spray. Spread mustard evenly over the non oil-side of each piece.

Place bread oil-side down into skillet, and layer with 2 ounces tempeh, 1 slice of Swiss cheese, and then sauerkraut. Place second piece of cheese on top of sauerkraut and top that with second piece of bread. For a lower calorie/lower fat version of this sandwich, omit the second piece of cheese — it just helps the sandwich stay together a bit better. Cook until toasted on one side, flip, and continue cooking until cheese melts. Or just cook on the panini press for about 3 to 4 minutes.

Feel free to add tomatoes, lettuce, or sprouts to this sandwich!

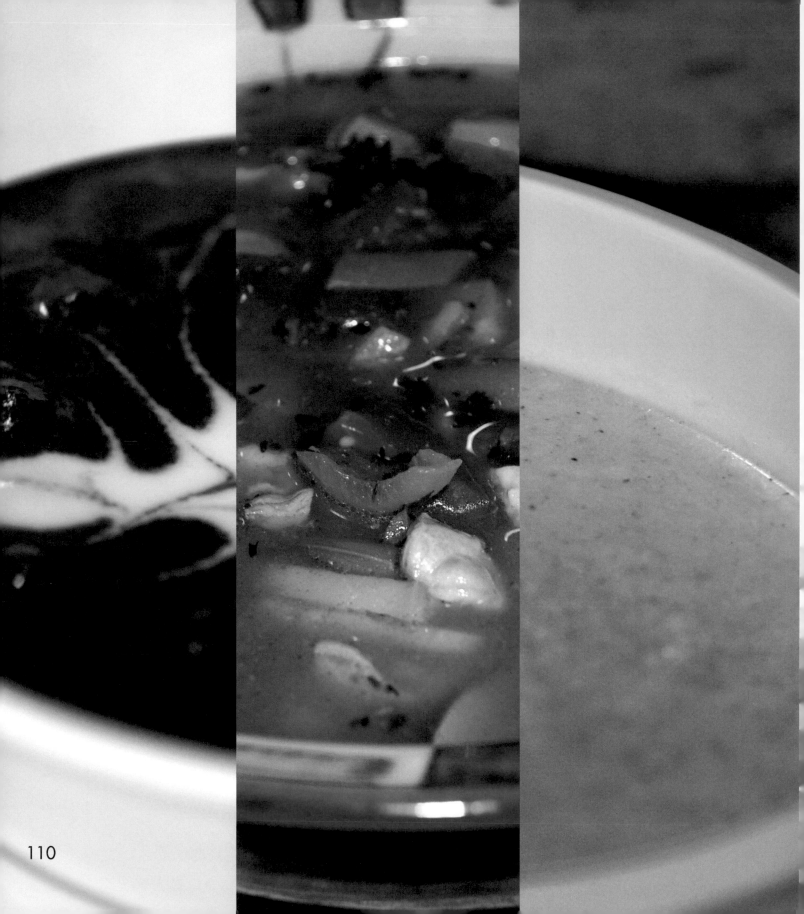

110

Worries go down better with soup. ~Jewish Proverb

Soups

Soup for Weight Loss?

Soup just may be a great bet when it comes to curbing your appetite – and we're not talking about the "cabbage soup diet" here. Penn State University performed a study where a group of women ate three different snacks that contained the same ingredients and same amount of calories: chicken rice casserole with a glass of water, or a soup made with the same ingredients. The soup curbed their appetite longest. All participants reported feeling less hunger and ate on average 80 calories less at their next meal.

The research leader said it appeared that soup offers a larger portion while sparing the calories. It appears that the mechanism is straight-forward. Your mouth likes the extra food; your brain likes the idea of having more; and now it appears that your stomach stays fuller longer than expected. All of these factors work together to help you feel more satisfied.

As a snack or a meal soup may be a super way to help you achieve greater satisfaction and your ideal weight.

Avocado Veggie Gazpacho

This twist on your standard gazpacho makes us very happy because we love avocados so much. You can adjust the spiciness by adding more or less jalapeno pepper. We like it to have a nice little kick – really gets the metabolism pumping

Serves 8

3 cups tomato-based vegetable
  juice (we use Very Veggie by Knudson)
2 cups tomatoes, seeded and
  diced (about 5 medium tomatoes)
1 tomatillo, diced
1 cup green bell pepper, diced
1 cup red onion, diced
1 medium cucumber, peeled,
  seeded, and diced
2 green onions, diced
1 tablespoon agave nectar or honey
2 medium avocados, pitted and diced
1 clove garlic, minced
1 tablespoon jalapeno chili pepper, minced
1 tablespoon red wine vinegar
1 tablespoon fresh lime juice
salt and pepper, to taste

Per Serving:
135 Calories;
8g Fat (1g sat);
3g Protein;
16g Carbohydrate;
4g Dietary Fiber;
0mg Cholesterol;
344mg Sodium.

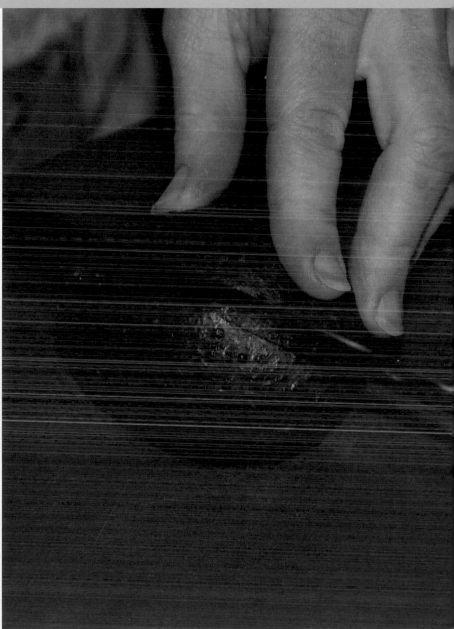

Combine all ingredients together in a large bowl or stockpot. Purée half of the ingredients in a blender or food processor and return to bowl with other diced ingredients. Use salt and pepper to taste. Garnish with cilantro and sour cream if desired. Serve chilled.

113

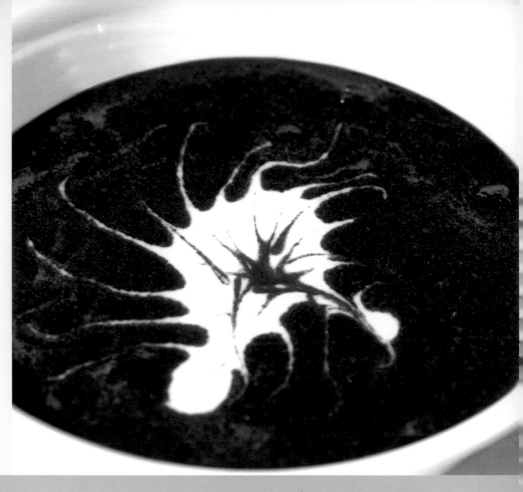

You can make this soup with fresh blueberries, however the frozen blueberries add a bit more liquid making it easier to purée. This is a fun, summery soup full of potent antioxidants and fiber.

Serves 3 to 4

Blue Soup

4 cups frozen blueberries
1 cup water
5 tablespoons sugar
½ lemon, sliced
1 cinnamon stick
½ teaspoon vanilla extract
3 tablespoons lowfat vanilla yogurt

Per Serving:
214 Calories;
2g Fat (trace sat fat);
2g Protein;
53g Carbohydrate;
8g Dietary Fiber;
1mg Cholesterol;
15mg Sodium.

Add all ingredients EXCEPT the yogurt to a large saucepan and heat over medium high until the sugar dissolves. Simmer for about 15 minutes. Remove lemon slices and cinnamon stick and purée half of the soup in blender or processor. Add puréed soup back to other ingredients and refrigerate until well chilled. Serve with one tablespoon yogurt on top.

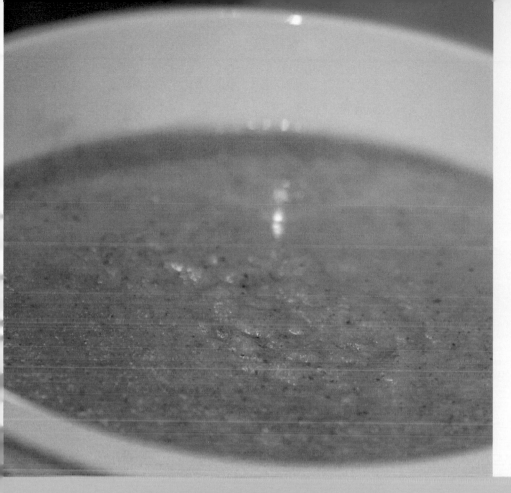

We love this soup – oh yes, you already know that because we love broccoli! This is a great accompaniment to any meal or as the main dish served in a large bowl with a nice piece of whole grain bread.

Serves 6

Per Serving:
143 Calories;
6g Fat (3g sat);
7g Protein;
17g Carbohydrate;
4g Dietary Fiber;
10mg Cholesterol;
638mg Sodium.

Cup of Greens

Heat water to boiling in 3-quart saucepan. Add broccoli flowerets and stalk pieces, celery, carrots, onion, and oats. Cover and return to a low boil. Simmer for about 10 minutes or until broccoli is tender (do not drain). Carefully place broccoli mixture in blender or food processor. Cover and blend on medium speed until smooth.

Melt butter in 3-quart saucepan over medium low heat. Stir in flour. Cook, stirring constantly, until mixture is smooth and bubbly; remove from heat. Stir broth into butter- flour mixture. Heat to boiling, stirring constantly for one minute. Reduce heat, stir in broccoli-vegetable mixture, salt, pepper and nutmeg. Return soup to a low simmer. Stir in milk – do not boil. Turn off heat or keep on low until ready to serve.

1½ pounds broccoli, chopped
2 cups water
1 large stalk celery (¾ cup), chopped
½ cup carrots, shredded
1 medium onion (½ cup), chopped
½ cup rolled oats
2 tablespoons butter
2 tablespoons potato flour or
   1 tablespoon corn starch mixed in
   1 tablespoon cool water
2 ½ cups chicken broth or vegetable broth
½ teaspoon salt
⅛ teaspoon pepper
Dash ground nutmeg
½ cup plain soy milk or lowfat milk

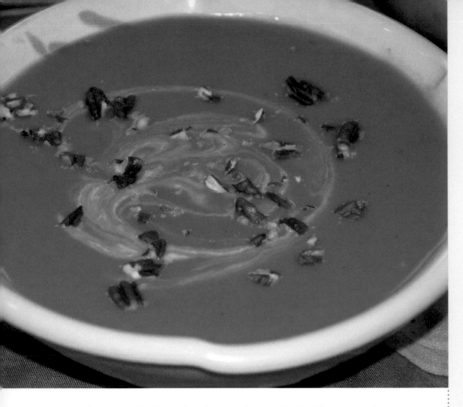

The spice that gives curry its bright yellow color is turmeric, the powdered dry rhizome (underground stem) of the Curcuma longa plant. Curcumin is a major anti-oxidant component of turmeric and has many fantastic qualities that benefit health. Curcumin has been shown to have anti-inflammatory properties and may decrease the risk of certain degenerative diseases including Alzheimer's. Turmeric and curcumin are once again in the news for their protective and therapeutic benefit against colon cancer. There are numerous test tube and animal studies and just a small handful of human trials demonstrating the potential effects of curcumin against colon cancer.

Heat butter and olive oil in large, deep sided skillet or stock pot over medium heat. Add onion, fresh ginger, and curry powder and sauté about five minutes. Add butternut squash and continue to cook about five minutes. Add roasted bell peppers, stirring once again to combine and cook for another five minutes.

Slowly add chicken broth to squash mixture and reduce heat to low. Cover and cook for about 20 minutes, until squash is soft.

In a blender, purée all ingredients until smooth. Depending on the size of your blender, you may need to do this in two batches. Add purée to soup pot. Heat again over low-medium heat. Stir in salt and pepper, to taste. Swirl in a teaspoon of yogurt or crème fraiche with each serving, as desired. Top with a teaspoon or two of toasted chopped pecans.

Per Serving:
308Calories;
11g Fat (2g sat);
12g Protein;
47g Carbohydrate;
8g Dietary Fiber;
5mg Cholesterol;
420mg Sodium.

Serves 6

1 tablespoon butter
1 tablespoon olive oil
2 tablespoons fresh ginger, minced
1 medium onion, chopped
1 to 2 tablespoons curry powder
1 medium butternut squash, peeled, seeded
    and cut into 1-inch cubes
1 cup roasted red or yellow bell peppers, chopped
4 cups low sodium chicken or vegetable broth
¼ teaspoon salt
¼ teaspoon white pepper

Sunset Soup

Black Diamond Chili

A spicy and hearty vegetarian alternative to traditional chili.

Serves 4

2 teaspoons olive oil
1 large onion, chopped (about a cup)
1 small green bell pepper,
 chopped (½ cup)
1 small red bell pepper, chopped
1 medium zucchini, chopped
1 cup chopped broccoli florets
2 cloves garlic, chopped
4 cups cooked black beans
2 (14½-ounce) cans tomatoes with diced
 green chilis, undrained
3 teaspoons chili powder
¼ cup sour cream, if desired
Salt and pepper to taste
Optional condiments: lowfat shredded
 cheese, minced onions, sour cream

For a meaty variation add browned ground
 turkey, beef or bison to this chili

Per Serving:
319 Calories;
7g Fat (2g sat);
17g Protein;
51g Carbohydrate;
18g Dietary Fiber;
6mg Cholesterol;
32mg Sodium.

Heat oil in a large soup or stock pot, over medium-high heat. Cook onion, peppers, zucchini, broccoli and garlic in oil, stirring frequently, until onion is tender. Stir in beans, tomatoes and chili powder; reduce heat. Cover and simmer 20 minutes. Add salt and pepper to taste. Serve with diced onions, shredded cheese and lowfat sour cream as desired.

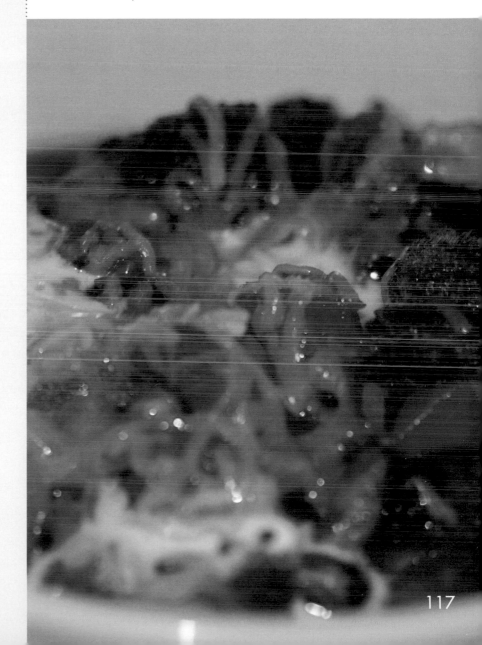

Cabin Fever Cure

Serves 6

1 tablespoon olive oil
1 medium onion, diced
1 large carrot, sliced
1 large stalk celery, sliced
¾ pound boneless skinless chicken breasts,
   cut into ¾-inch cubes
1½ cups diced tomatoes, 1 15-ounce can
½ cup chopped zucchini
½ cup green beans, chopped
6 cups reduced-sodium chicken broth
1 teaspoon dried thyme leaves
2 tablespoons chopped fresh parsley
salt and pepper (optional)

Add olive oil, onions, carrots, and celery to a large stockpot. Heat over medium-high and stir until onions are translucent. Add chicken and continue to cook until chicken is nearly cooked. Add diced tomatoes, zucchini, green beans, broth, and thyme. Bring to a boil, then reduce heat to low and cover. Cook for an additional 10 minutes, then add fresh parsley and season with salt and pepper.

Per Serving:
160 Calories;
3g Fat (1g sat);
25g Protein;
8g Carbohydrate;
2g Dietary Fiber;
33mg Cholesterol;
571mg Sodium.

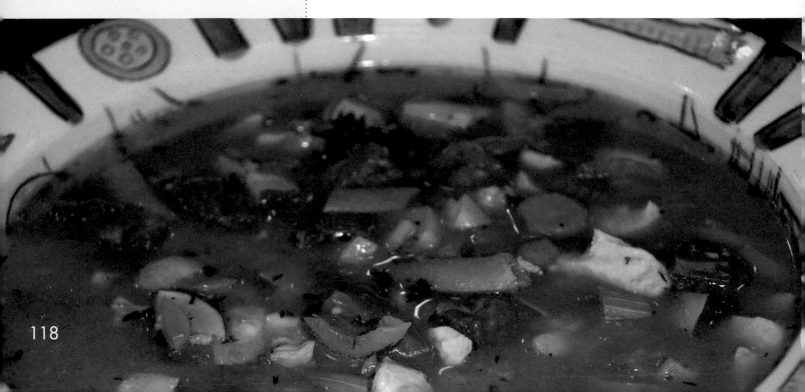

Strawberry Soup

Combine all ingredients in blender or food processor and blend until you attain desired consistency. Keep chilled until ready to serve. For a thicker, colder soup, use frozen strawberries and a good blender! Serve with a slice of kiwi and a sprig of mint on top.

Per Serving
(about ¾ cup):
122 Calories; 1g Fat
(0g Sat); 7g Protein;
24g Carbohydrate;
2g Dietary Fiber;
2mg Cholesterol;
88mg Sodium.

A creamy alternative to blueberry soup! You can also turn this into a fabulous frozen yogurt if you have an ice-cream maker – just add everything to the ice cream maker and follow the manufacturer's directions, then freeze and enjoy (or make popsicles out of it!)

Serves 4 to 5

2 cups plain nonfat yogurt
2 cups sliced fresh strawberries
½ tablespoon orange juice
2 tablespoons honey
1 tablespoon fresh lime juice

GARNISH:
mint sprigs
kiwi slices

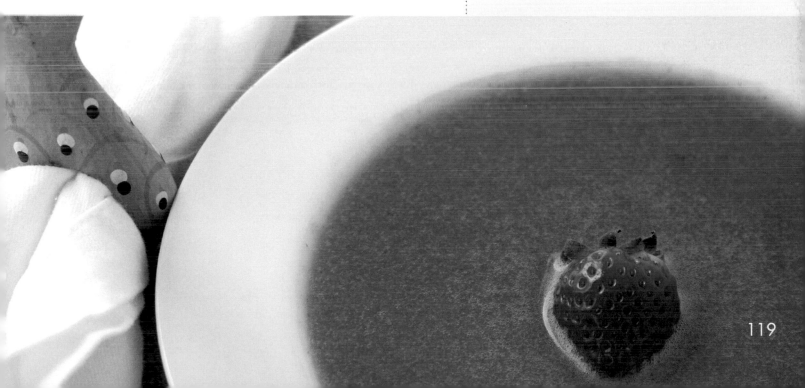

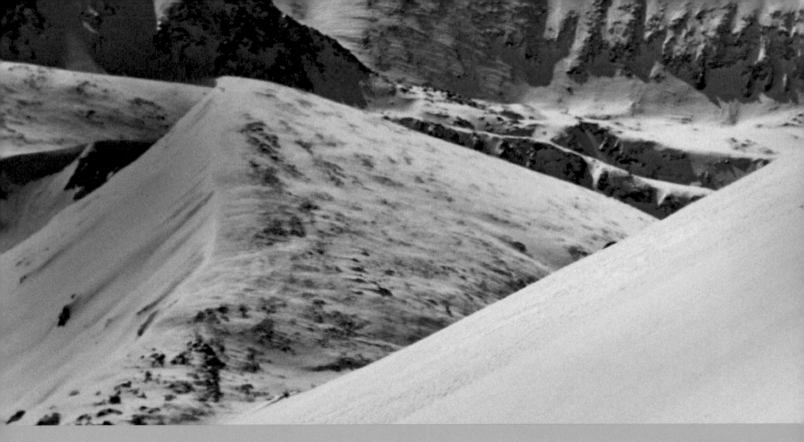

Warming Hut Welcome

Add olive oil to medium size soup or stock pot and heat over medium heat. Add sausage slices and sauté for 5 minutes or until slightly browned. Add vegetables (shallots through potatoes) and continue to sauté for an additional 5 minutes. Add flour and cook for 2 more minutes. Add chicken broth, and optional salt and pepper and stir until smooth. Simmer for 30 minutes or until potatoes are soft. Garnish with green onions and sour cream (or yogurt) if desired.

Per Serving:
321 Calories;
12g Fat (3 g sat);
15g Protein;
41g Carbohydrate;
7g Dietary Fiber;
166mg Cholesterol;
593mg Sodium.

Serves 4

2 teaspoons olive oil
12 ounces chicken and apple sausages, sliced into
  ⅛" thick slices (vegetarians may substitute soy
  sausage or crumbled tempeh)
½ cup shallots, chopped fine
½ cup celery, chopped
2 cups peeled, diced sweet potatoes or yellow potatoes
2 tablespoons flour (we use potato flour)
4 cups low sodium chicken (or vegetable) broth
salt and pepper to taste
Green onions, garnish
lowfat sour cream or plain yogurt

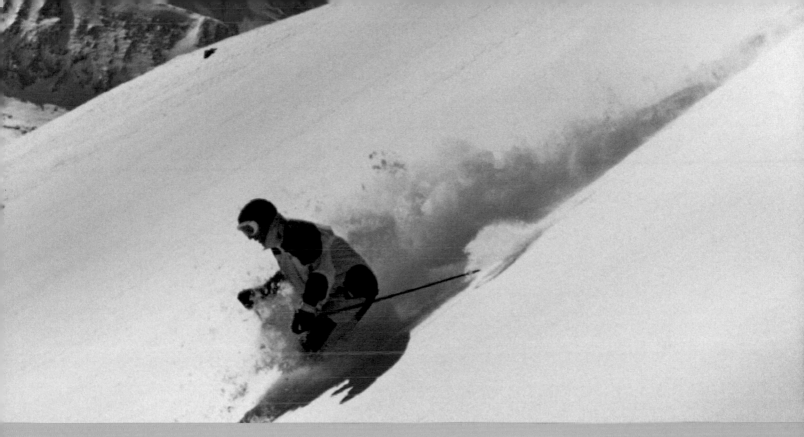

Powder Day Chili

Serves 8

1 tablespoon olive oil
1 pound ground turkey breast
1 cup onion (1 medium), chopped
1 cup diced green chiles
1 clove garlic, finely chopped
3 cups low sodium chicken broth
1 tablespoon chili powder
1 teaspoon cumin powder
½ teaspoon salt
¼ teaspoon black pepper
2 cups diced tomatoes (no salt)
1 (15-ounce) can (low salt) black beans, drained
1 (15-ounce) can (low salt) pinto beans, drained

Heat oil in 3-quart saucepan over medium-high heat. Cook turkey, onion, green chiles and garlic in oil, stirring occasionally, until turkey is no longer pink in center and onion is tender.

Stir in remaining ingredients. Heat to simmer; reduce heat. Cover and simmer 30 minutes, stirring occasionally.

Per Serving:
239 Calories; 3g Fat
(12.0% calories from fat); 25g
Protein; 28g Carbohydrate; 2g
Dietary Fiber; 65mg Cholesterol;
883mg Sodium** (sodium
content is dependent on type of
broth used and additional
salt added).

121

Snow Day soup

Serves 5 to 6

½ cup burdock root, peeled and sliced into thin slices
½ cup carrots sliced into ¼ inch slices
½ cup beets, well scrubbed and sliced into ½ inch pieces
½ cup cabbage thinly sliced
½ cup diced red onion
2 leeks, well-rinsed and sliced into ¼ inch slivers
½ cup shiitake mushrooms, sliced
2 cloves garlic, minced
1 tablespoon minced fresh ginger
2 tablespoons extra-virgin olive oil
5 cups chicken or vegetable broth (or water)
2 tablespoons light miso
2 scallions, minced
2 tablespoons fresh cilantro

Per Serving:
169 Calories;
5g Fat (1g sat);
4g Protein;
27g Carbohydrate;
4g Dietary Fiber;
0mg Cholesterol;
665mg Sodium.

Sauté burdock, carrots, cabbage, beets, leeks, onion, shiitake, garlic, and ginger in olive oil (in large stock pot) for 10 minutes.

Add broth or water and bring to a low boil. Lower heat, cover and simmer for 20 minutes or until vegetables are tender. Dilute miso in small amount of hot broth and add to soup. Turn off heat, add scallions, cover and let stand for 5 minutes. Top with fresh cilantro.

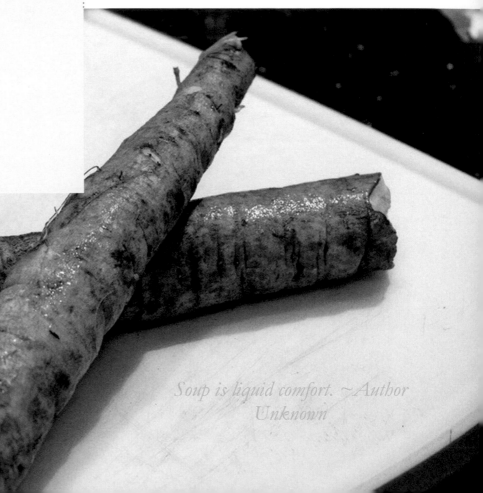

Soup is liquid comfort. ~Author Unknown

122

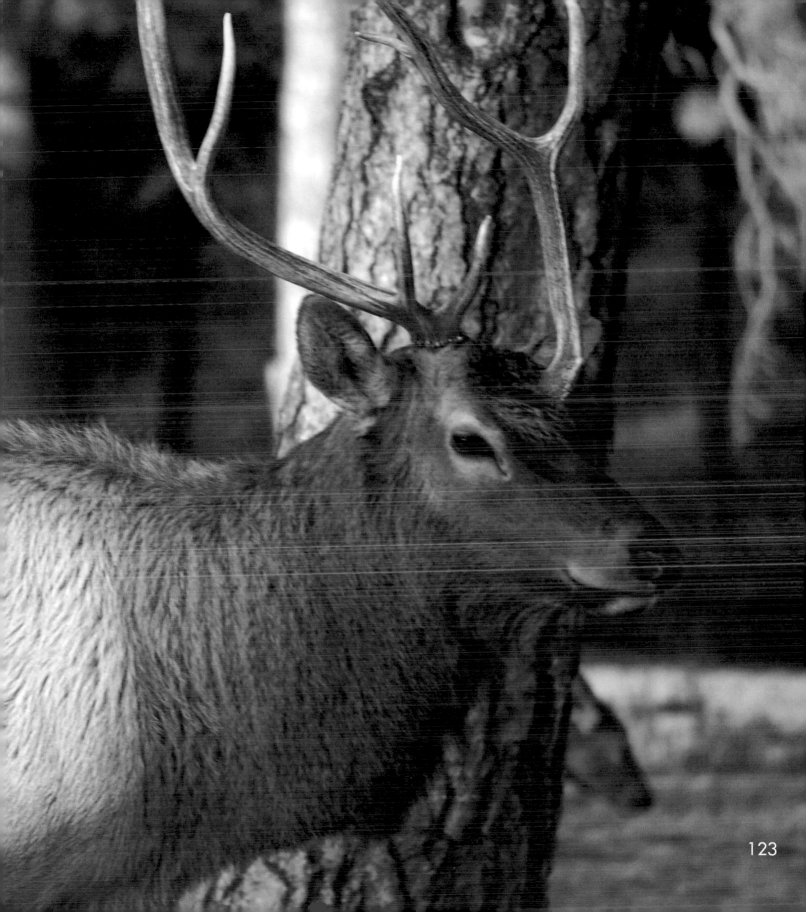

The Sweet Sweet Potato

Sweet potatoes certainly deserve more attention than just a once a year Thanksgiving dinner kind of food. There are many reasons to choose sweet potatoes year round. Sweet potatoes actually aren't even in the potato family. They are an edible root, rather than an edible tuber (the potato is a tuber). Sweet potatoes are native to the United States and were a highly valued food by Native Americans.

Sweet potatoes not only taste great, but their nutritional content is pretty awesome. Four ounces of baked sweet potato (about 1 medium sweet potato, with skin), contains over 3 ½ grams of fiber and 12 milligrams of beta carotene (that's an entire day's worth of this nutrient!). Beta-carotene is primarily responsible for giving sweet potato its orange colored sweet flesh. Sweet potatoes are also an excellent source of vitamins C, B6, biotin, B5, E, and the minerals iron and potassium. Sweet potatoes may offer significant antioxidant qualities. Sweet potatoes are a much better choice for diabetics than regular potatoes as sweet potatoes may help stabilize blood sugar.

The skin of sweet potatoes is edible. Like any vegetable, it should be scrubbed and washed well and you should look for any bruises, spots, mold or decay. You want to avoid those and if the pickings are slim, then you can cut those areas away. You want the potato to be firm and smooth. Don't use it, if it is mushy or overly bruised.

It's easy to incorporate sweet potatoes into the diet. You can bake them like you would a white potato and serve them plain or you can cut it up into small cubes and roast in the oven with a little olive oil and fresh rosemary. You can also bake the potatoes and then scoop out the flesh and use to make a great soup – especially puréed with a little vegetable or chicken broth, a little ginger, a cooked carrot or two and a granny smith apple. Top that with a dollup of sour cream or crème fraiche and you've got a delightful fall soup. You can also add cubed sweet potato to stir-frys. One of our favorite things to do is to bake the sweet potato then scoop out the flesh and mash it with a little ghee (clarified butter), pumpkin pie spice, and a tiny bit of maple syrup.

Life expectancy would grow by leaps and bounds if green vegetables smelled as good as bacon. ~Doug Larson

Sides

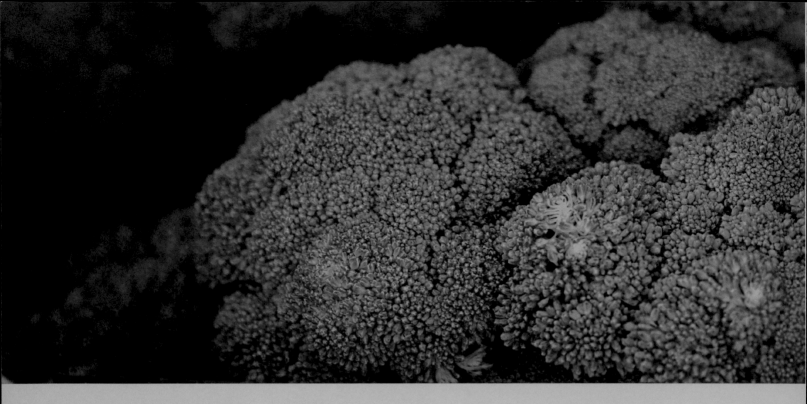

Evergreen Risotto

Combine oil and butter in a large saucepan and heat over medium. Add onion and garlic, and sauté 3 to 4 minutes until onions are softened. Stir in rice, salt and pepper, and cook 1 minute more.

Add 1 cup broth to the saucepan, and cook, stirring constantly, about 3 minutes, or until most of the broth has been absorbed. Stir in another cup of broth, and cook, stirring occasionally to prevent sticking, until liquid is absorbed. Repeat in ½ cup increments until you have ½ cup stock left. Add broccoli and last ½ cup of broth; cook 4 minutes more, or until broth is absorbed and broccoli is tender. Fold in cheese and lemon zest. Serve immediately.

Per Serving:
303 Calories;
8g Fat (3g sat);
15g Protein;
43g Carbohydrate;
1g Dietary Fiber;
12mg Cholesterol;
792mg Sodium.

Serves 4

1 tablespoon olive oil
1 tablespoon butter
1 small onion, diced
2 cloves garlic cloves, minced
1 cup uncooked arborio rice, for more fiber
   substitute short grain brown rice
½ teaspoon salt
¼ teaspoon black pepper
3 cups low sodium chicken broth
1 cup broccoli florets, finely chopped
¼ cup grated fresh Parmesan cheese, or Romano
1 tablespoon lemon zest

Wildflower Sauté

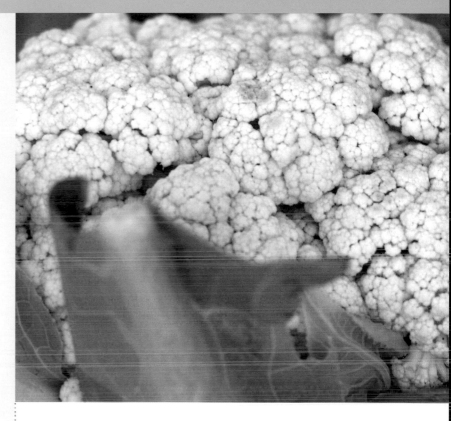

This is a wonderfully healthful side dish that can accompany just about any meal. The phytonutrient combination of cauliflower and turmeric benefits our health. Cauliflower, like other cruciferous vegetables, contains glucosinolates and thiocyanates, which are compounds that may prevent cancer. Turmeric has long been recognized as a powerful anti-inflammatory agent in both Chinese and Indian systems of medicine, and modern scientific research continues to reinforce the benefits of this tasty spice. One serving of this dish also provides 181% of the daily value (DV) for vitamin C, 46% DV for vitamin K, and 33% DV for folate. Enjoy!

Serves 4

1 pound cauliflower (or about 4 cups cauliflower florets)
5 tablespoons low-sodium chicken or vegetable broth
1 teaspoon turmeric (or use curry powder)

Dressing
2 tablespoons extra virgin olive oil
2 teaspoons lemon juice
1 medium garlic clove, minced
sea salt and pepper to taste

Per Serving
(1 cup): 90 Calories;
7g Fat (1g sat);
3g Protein;
6g Carbohydrate;
2g Dietary Fiber;
0mg Cholesterol;
70mg Sodium.

Rinse cauliflower well and cut into florets, rinsing again to get any "critters" out of the nooks and crannies (this is usually the case with organic cauliflower).

Heat 5 tablespoons of broth in a stainless steel skillet over medium heat. When broth begins to steam, add cauliflower and turmeric and cover. For al dente cauliflower, cook for no more than 5 minutes.

In a medium size bowl or mason jar, whisk together olive oil, lemon juice, minced garlic, salt and pepper.

Drain cauliflower from broth and transfer to a bowl. Toss the cauliflower with the dressing until evenly coated.

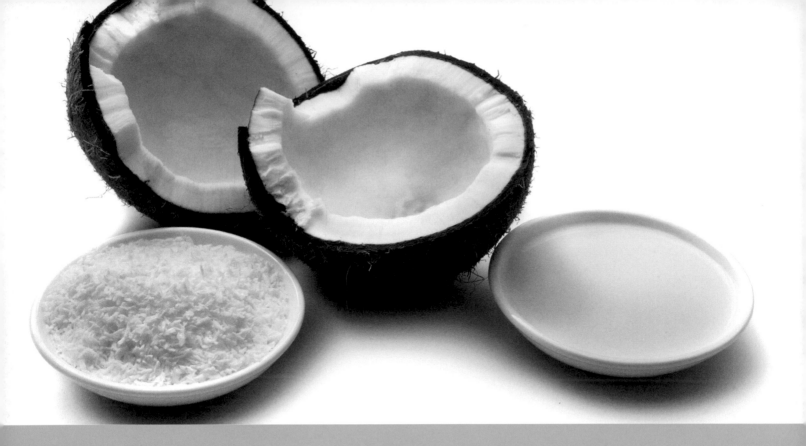

Coconut Rice

Rinse and drain rice. Combine rice with chicken broth and coconut milk and bring to a low boil. Reduce heat and cover. Stir occasionally. Cook for 40 minutes, then remove cover and stir in scallions, lime zest, and shredded coconut meat. If all the liquid has cooked off, add a little bit more coconut milk (or broth for less of the coconut flavor) and cover and cook for another 5 minutes. Allow to sit covered for 5 minutes before fluffing with a fork. Serve warm.

Serves 4

1 cup brown rice, medium-grain
1 cup low sodium chicken broth
1 cup light coconut milk
2 medium scallions, chopped
1 teaspoon lime zest
1 tablespoon shredded coconut meat

Per Serving:
225 Calories;
5g Fat (2g sat);
7g Protein;
40g Carbohydrate;
1g Dietary Fiber;
0mg Cholesterol;
148mg Sodium.

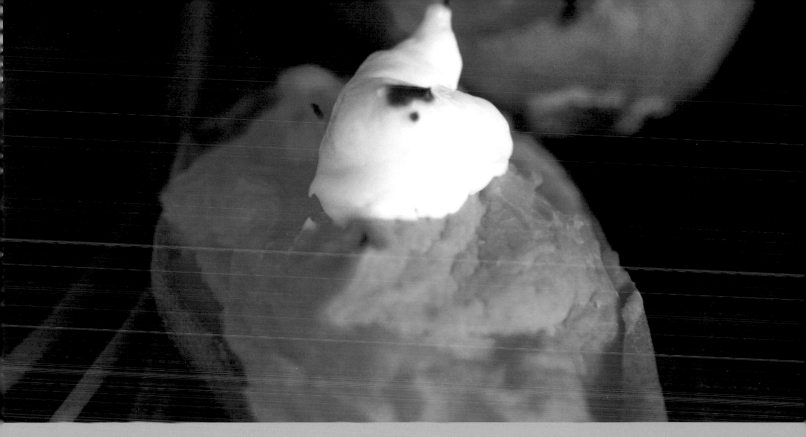

Sweet Spuds

These are just heavenly. Sweet potatoes are part of the favorite food club in our house.

Serves 4

3 medium sweet potatoes or yams (of equal size)
3 tablespoons fresh orange juice
3 ounces Neufchatel cheese softened and divided
1 teaspoon fresh chives
salt and white pepper, to taste

Per Serving:
163 Calories;
5g Fat (3g sat);
2g Protein;
2g Carbohydrate;
3 Dietary Fiber;
16mg Cholesterol;
85mg Sodium

Preheat oven to 375°F. Bake sweet potatoes until a fork can be inserted easily, about 50 minutes to an hour. Cut potatoes in half lengthwise and scrape pulp out of skins, leaving about ⅛ inch of potato lining the skin.

In a food processor, combine cooked pulp, orange juice, and 2 ounces of Neufchatel. Purée just until mixed. Add salt and white pepper to taste.

Refill 4 sweet potato skins with purée. Toss out the extra skins. Heat through for 15 minutes at 375°F. Preheat broiler. Spoon remaining Neufchatel on top of each potato. Place underneath broiler just until Neufchatel begins to brown. Watch carefully to avoid burning.

Garnish with fresh chopped chives.

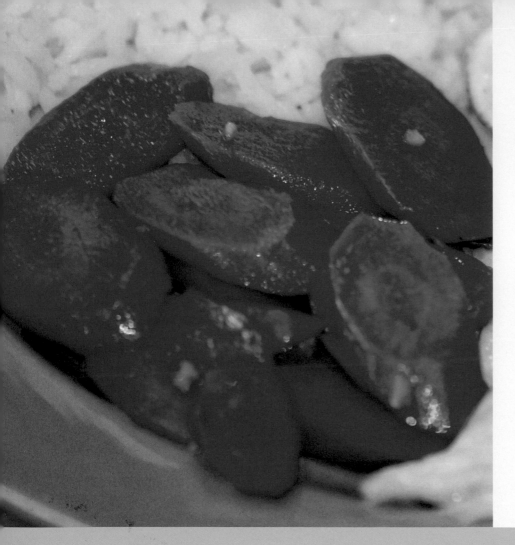

If you think you don't like cooked carrots, you have to give this recipe a try, because we think you'll reconsider. Carrots are an amazing source of antioxidant vitamins and minerals. Carrots are one of the vegetables we recommend you always buy organic. They have been listed among the "dirty dozen" of foods on which pesticide residues have been most frequently found.

Serves 6

Gingered Carrots

Steam carrots on stovetop or microwave until barely tender; drain. While carrots are cooking, combine canola oil and ginger in a small saucepan. Cook over medium heat for about 2 minutes. Add maple syrup and orange juice, stirring constantly, until sauce thickens.
Cook about a minute, then remove from heat and stir in carrots. Cover and let sit about 5 minutes before serving. Serve warm.

Per Serving:
98 Calories;
5g Fat (trace sat);
1g Protein;
14g Carbohydrate;
2g Dietary Fiber;
0mg Cholesterol;
26mg Sodium.

6 medium carrots – thinly sliced
 (3 cups)
2 tablespoons canola oil
1 teaspoon fresh ginger, minced
3 tablespoons maple syrup
1 tablespoon orange juice

130

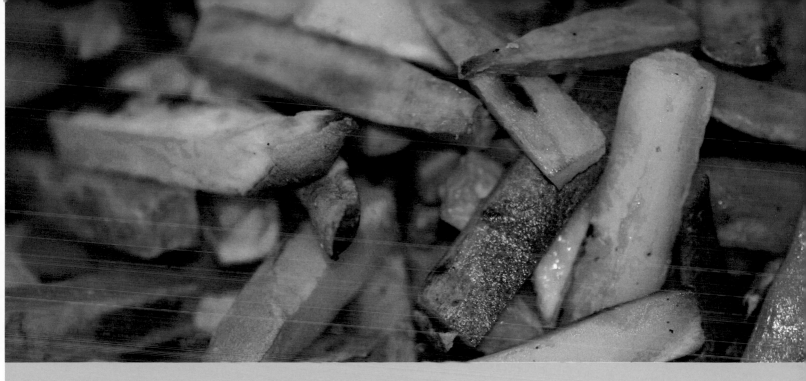

Fancy Fries

Preheat oven to 375°F. Line baking pan with parchment or aluminum foil. Alternatively you can just spray the pan with cooking oil spray.

Scrub and wash potatoes well. No need to peel potatoes. Cut potatoes into thin strips and place in a large bowl. Add oil and sprinkle with salt and pepper.

Carefully place potatoes on prepared baking pan. Bake for about 30 to 40 minutes, turning so that all sides cook and brown equally. Fries are done with they reach desired consistency. We like them soft in the middle and slightly crispy on the outside.

Per Serving:
187 Calories;
4g Fat (1g sat);
2g Protein;
37g Carbohydrate;
5g Dietary Fiber;
0mg Cholesterol;
250mg Sodium.

These "Fries" are actually baked, not fried. As a result you'll get tons of flavor without the fat or trans fat that usually comes along with traditional fries. Sweet potatoes are about the most nutritious vegetables around. They are loaded with beta-carotene, vitamin C, fiber, iron, vitamin B6, manganese and potassium. Choose sweet potatoes and yams that are firm without any bruises, soft spots or cracks.

Serves 4

2 medium sweet potato
2 medium yams
1 tablespoon olive oil
½ teaspoon sea salt

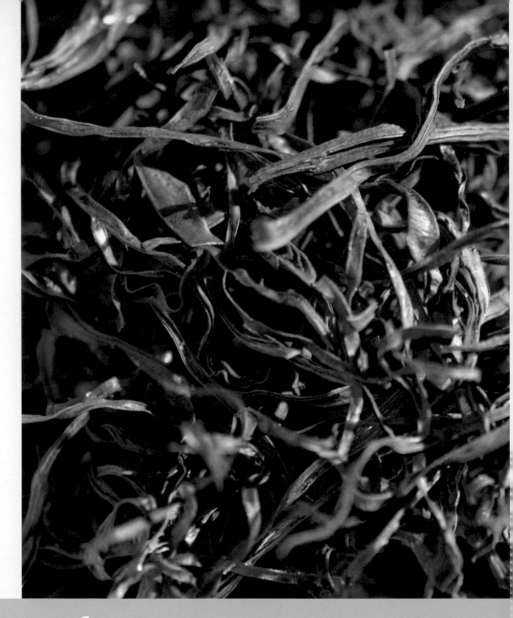

Arame is a sea vegetable (aka seaweed), that contains essential minerals and trace minerals as well as vitamins B1, B2, B6, niacin, vitamin C, B12 (rare in vegetables), and beta-carotene. Kale is the Rouse House vegetable of choice (along with broccoli) and it's health benefits go on and on. Call it a sauté, call it a salad, this dish is over-the-top good for you.

Serves 4

Per Serving:
186 Calories;
10g Fat (1g sat);
8g Protein;
21g Carbohydrate;
5g Dietary Fiber;
0mg Cholesterol;
194mg Sodium.

Sea of Greens

2 tablespoons olive oil
½ cup aramé seaweed
(soaked in pure warm water 20 minutes)
1½ pounds kale or chard, trimmed and
*   cut into pieces (1 inch)*
½ cup onion, diced
¼ cup low sodium vegetable broth
2 tablespoons toasted sesame seeds

Add olive oil and onion to a nonstick skillet and heat over medium high heat, stirring onion with wooden spatula to keep from browning. Drain aramé. Add kale and pre-soaked aramé to skillet and stir-fry for about 2 minutes. Add vegetable broth, cover and cook over medium for an additional 4 or 5 minutes. Turn off heat, add toasted sesame seeds and toss.

Fungus Among Us

The flavors in this dish are delicious. If you don't have walnut oil, feel free to substitute olive oil.

Serves 4

½ bunch green onions
1 large portobello mushroom cap, sliced
2 tablespoons walnut oil, divided
¾ pounds asparagus spears
2 teaspoons balsamic vinegar
½ teaspoon sea salt
½ teaspoon black pepper
¼ teaspoon basil

Toss green onions and Portobello mushrooms with 1 tablespoon of the walnut oil. Spread into baking dish and roast at 450°F for about 10 minutes. Toss the asparagus with the remaining oil and add to the roasting pan. Sprinkle the balsamic vinegar, salt, pepper, and basil over the top. Roast for another 10 minutes or until the veggies are crisp and delicious.

Per Serving:
80 Calories;
7g Fat (1g sat);
2g Protein;
4g Carbohydrate;
1g Dietary Fiber;
0mg Cholesterol;
238mg Sodium

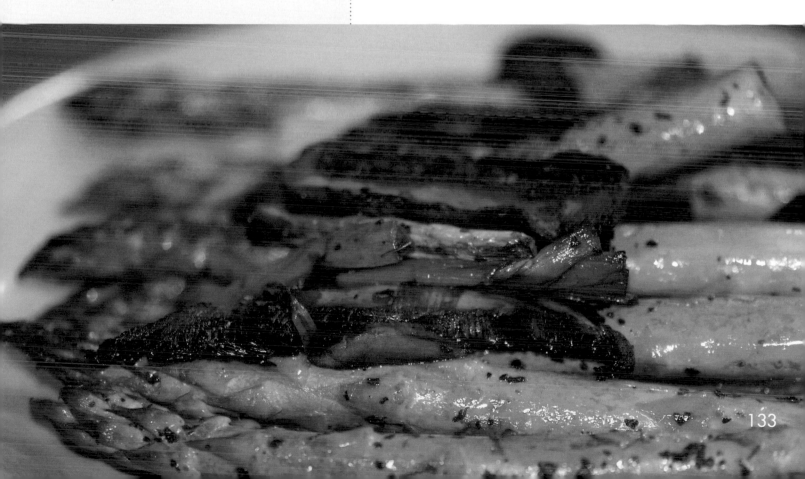

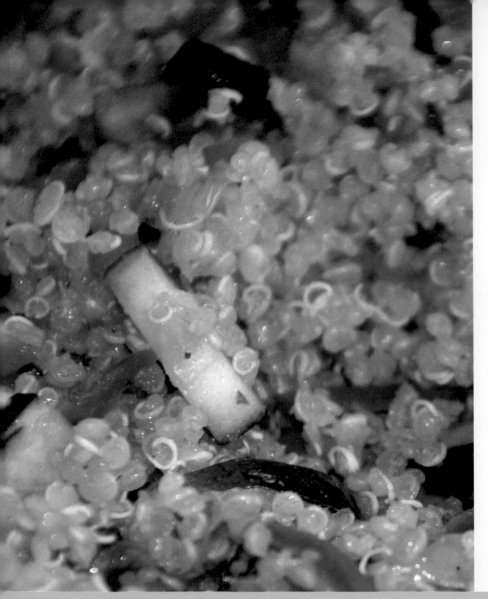

Quinoa (pronounced Keen-wah), is a relative of spinach and Swiss chard. It is a nutty seed-like "ancient grain" that is high in complete protein, magnesium, manganese, iron, tryptophan and fiber. Quinoa is a great choice for vegan vegetarians due to its unique complete protein and it is naturally gluten-free. We usually rinse quinoa two or three times to remove the soapy saponin residue that can coat the seed.

Serves 4

Per Serving:
235 Calories;
6g Fat (1g sat);
13g Protein;
35g Carbohydrate;
6g Dietary Fiber;
0mg Cholesterol;
306mg Sodium

Quinoa Pilaf

Sauté vegetables and garlic in olive oil until tender-crisp.

Add broth to vegetables. Bring to a rolling boil.

Add quinoa to vegetables and broth and stir. Cover and reduce heat to low. Simmer until all liquid is absorbed and the grains are fluffy, about 15 minutes.

1 tablespoon olive oil
4 scallions, thinly sliced
½ cup sliced fresh mushrooms
1 garlic clove, minced
½ cup chopped zucchini
½ cup chopped red bell pepper
¼ cup shredded carrots
2 ¼ cups low sodium vegetable broth
1 cup quinoa, rinsed and drained

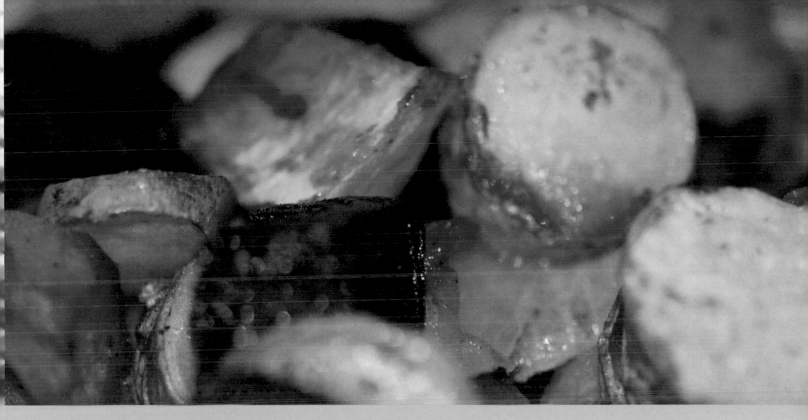

Roasted Roots

Serves 4

4 medium red potatoes, well scrubbed and cubed
3 medium beets, well scrubbed, peeled, and cubed
2 medium carrots, scrubbed and chopped into ½ inch rounds
1 medium red onion, sliced in half then quartered
2 large portobello mushroom caps, sliced
1 tablespoon olive oil
¼ teaspoon salt
⅛ teaspoon black pepper
1 teaspoon fresh rosemary, chopped

Per Serving:
188 Calories;
4g Fat (1g sat);
5g Protein;
36g Carbohydrate;
6g Dietary Fiber;
0mg Cholesterol;
203mg Sodium.

Preheat oven to 450°F. Move oven rack to position second from the top in oven.

In a large bowl, combine vegetables (potatoes through mushroom caps). Drizzle with olive oil and season with salt, pepper, and rosemary. Toss well to combine.

Line a large baking tray (you may need two trays) with aluminum foil. Spray foil with cooking spray. Arrange vegetable mixture on foil so that nothing overlaps.

Place tray(s) in the oven to roast for 30 minutes. Gently push the vegetables around on the tray with a spatula and roast for another 3 minutes or until the root veggies are fork tender.

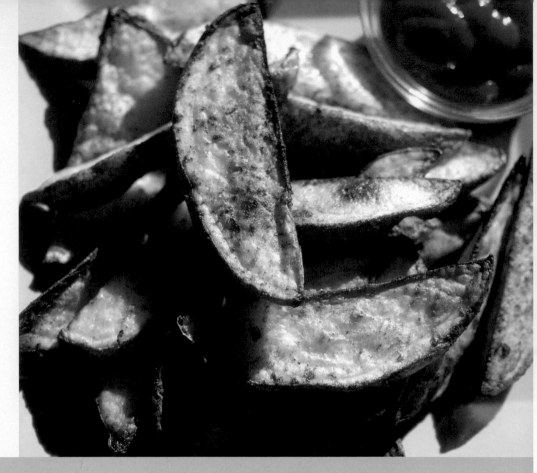

Another twist on your typical "fry." You can substitute sweet potatoes in lieu of the russet potatoes.

Serves 4

Spicy Spuds

2 medium russet potatoes (¾ pound)
(or sweet potatoes)
1 tablespoon olive oil
¼ teaspoon cinnamon
⅛ teaspoon red pepper
¼ teaspoon garlic powder
¼ teaspoon sea salt
⅛ teaspoon pepper

Per Serving:
198 Calories;
7g Fat (1g sat);
2g Protein;
32g Carbohydrate;
4g Dietary Fiber;
0mg Cholesterol;
252mg Sodium.

Preheat oven to 450°F. Line jelly roll pan with foil or parchment paper and spray lightly with cooking spray. Cut potatoes into ½-inch wedges. Combine spices with oil in a large plastic zipper baggie and add potatoes. Make sure the baggie is sealed and shake well until potatoes are well coated. Arrange potatoes in single layer in prepared pan.

Bake uncovered 25 to 30 minutes, turning occasionally, until potatoes are golden brown and tender when pierced with fork.

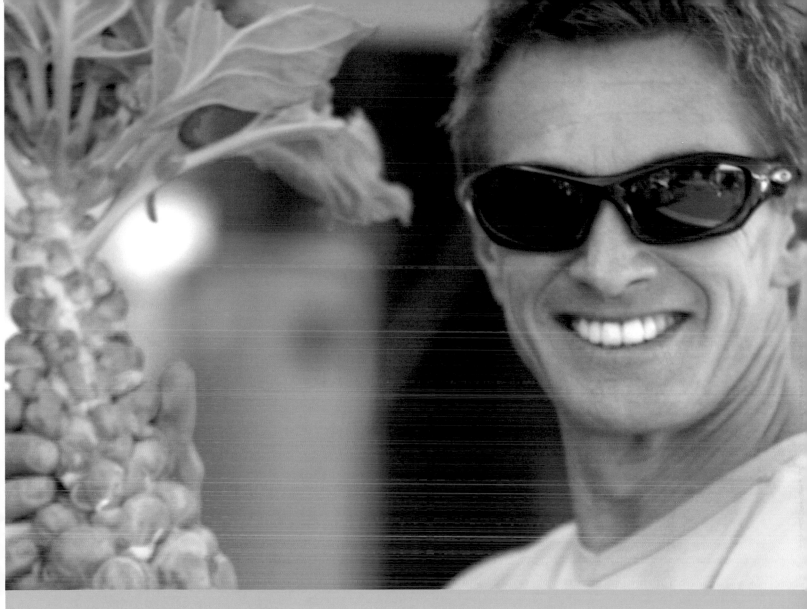

Super Sprouts

Rinse sprouts and remove discolored leaves. Cut sprouts in half and slice thin lengthwise. Add butter and olive oil to a heavy skillet and heat over moderately high heat until butter is melted. Add shallots and Brussels Sprouts and stir-fry until tender and lightly browned, about 8 minutes. Remove from heat and add to a large bowl. Drizzle fresh lime juice on top, season with sea salt and pepper and toss. Serve warm.

Per Serving:
133 Calories;
10g Fat (3g sat);
4g Protein;
10g Carbohydrate;
4g Dietary Fiber;
8mg Cholesterol;
27mg Sodium.

Serves 4

1 pound Brussels sprouts, thinly sliced
1 tablespoon unsalted butter
2 tablespoons olive oil
2 large shallots, thinly sliced
2 teaspoons fresh lime juice
sea salt and pepper to taste

137

Kale is loaded with phytonutrients that assist the body in detoxification. It is a rich source of fiber and vitamin K, which is essential for our bones and blood.

Serves 4

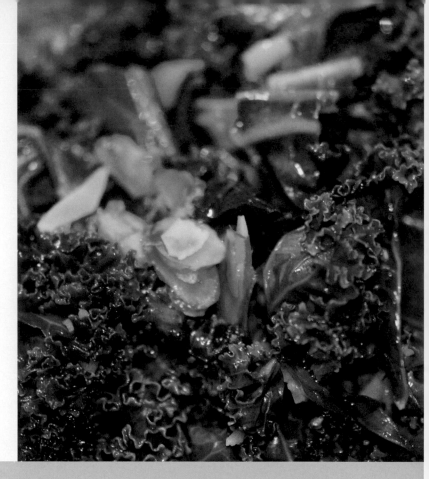

Crunchy Kale

1½ *pounds kale or chard, trimmed and cut into*
  1-inch pieces
2 *tablespoons olive oil*
1 *clove garlic, minced*
1 *teaspoon fresh ginger, peeled and minced*
¼ *cup slivered almonds*
2 *tablespoons low sodium chicken or vegetable broth*
1 *tablespoon tamari soy sauce*

Per Serving:
204 Calories;
13g Fat (2g sat);
8g Protein;
19g Carbohydrate;
4g Dietary Fiber;
0mg Cholesterol;
342mg Sodium

Heat a large nonstick skillet over medium high heat. Add olive oil, garlic and ginger and sauté for about 30 seconds. Add almonds and stir-fry about one minute. Add kale, broth and tamari soy sauce. Stir-fry about 5 minutes or until kale is wilted but not soggy.

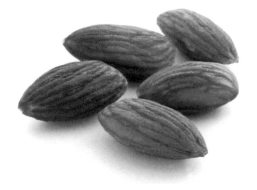

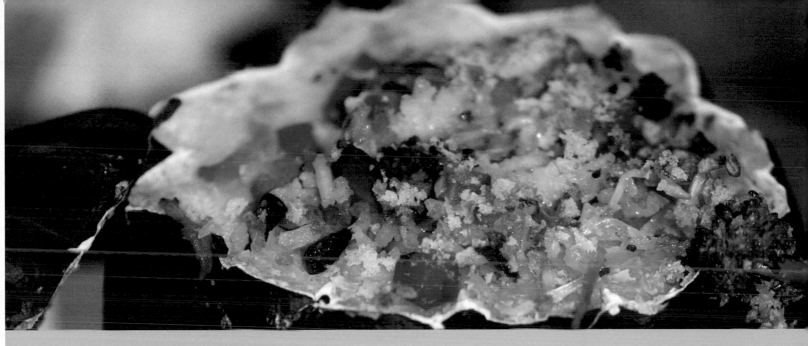

San Luis Squash

Preheat oven to 375°F. Take a small slice off the bottom so that the squash is able to sit in a pan without tilting over. Slice off the top of the squash, about ½ inch from the top. Remove the seeds and scrape out excess stringyness. Set squash in a large baking dish or roasting pan lined with parchment paper or aluminum foil. Bake the squash for about 20 minutes and remove from oven.

In a large skillet heat olive oil or butter over medium high. Add chopped onion and saute for about five minutes, stirring frequently. Add bell pepper, broccoli and carrots and stir for another three or four minutes. Stir in chopped spinach and stir another minute until spinach is wilted. Turn off heat and stir in rice, olives, Bragg's, oregano, and pepper.

Place ¼ of the mixture (about ¾ cup) in the cavity of the squash. Sprinkle top with bread crumbs. Bake for about 35 minutes on lower oven rack until squash is soft and top is lightly browned.

Serves 4

4 acorn squash
1 tablespoon olive oil, or butter
½ cup chopped onion
½ medium red bell pepper, chopped
1 cup broccoli florets
½ cup shredded carrots
2 cups chopped spinach
1½ cups cooked brown rice
2 tablespoons kalamata olives, pitted and chopped
1 tablespoon Bragg's Liquid Aminos
1 teaspoon oregano
¼ teaspoon pepper
4 tablespoons bread crumbs, optional

Per Serving:
359 Calories;
7g Fat (1g sat);
8g Protein;
74g Carbohydrate;
10g Dietary Fiber;
0mg Cholesterol;
449mg Sodium.

139

Front Range Stuffed Peppers

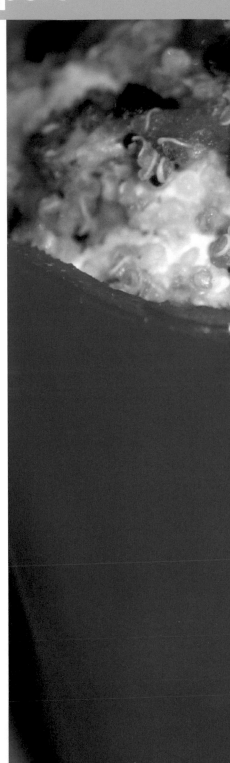

Rinse the quinoa well by pouring it into a fine colander or strainer and run water through it until the water runs clear. Gently tap the sides of the strainer to allow any excess water to escape. Then combine quinoa with 2 cups of water in a medium size pot and bring to a boil. Once it reaches boiling, lower the heat, cover and simmer 10 to 12 minutes, until all liquid is absorbed and the grains are fluffy.

Slice the tops off the bell peppers about ½ inch down from the stem. Rinse the bell peppers and remove the seeds and ribs from the inside of the peppers. From the tops that were cut off, cut off the bell pepper surrounding the stem - make sure it is well rinsed and then dice and add to a medium size bowl.

Fill a large pot with water and heat until boiling. Once the water reaches boiling, submerge the larger bell peppers into the water and allow to simmer for about five minutes. Remove to a large colander in the sink to allow to drain (or you can set them upside down on a paper towel or two).

In a large skillet, heat olive oil over medium high heat. Add onions, garlic and sausage and stir-fry for about 5 minutes. Add the reserved chopped bell peppers and broccoli and cook another five minutes. Add pine nuts and cumin and stir for about a minute and then add the diced zucchini, chopped spinach, fresh oregano, and sea salt. Stir for another 3 minutes and then add the cooked quinoa and the feta.

Preheat your oven to 425°F. Set the bell peppers in a large rectangular baking dish that has been coated with cooking spray or lined with parchment paper. Fill each bell pepper with the quinoa and veggie mixture. After all the peppers have been filled sprinkle the remaining feta over the tops. Bake for 25 minutes (or if you have prepared the peppers ahead of time and they have been refrigerated, allow about 30 minutes for cooking.)

You will likely have extra quinoa-vegetable filling leftover. Save it for another meal or make the peppers your main dish and serve additional quinoa filling around the pepper in a shallow salad bowl.

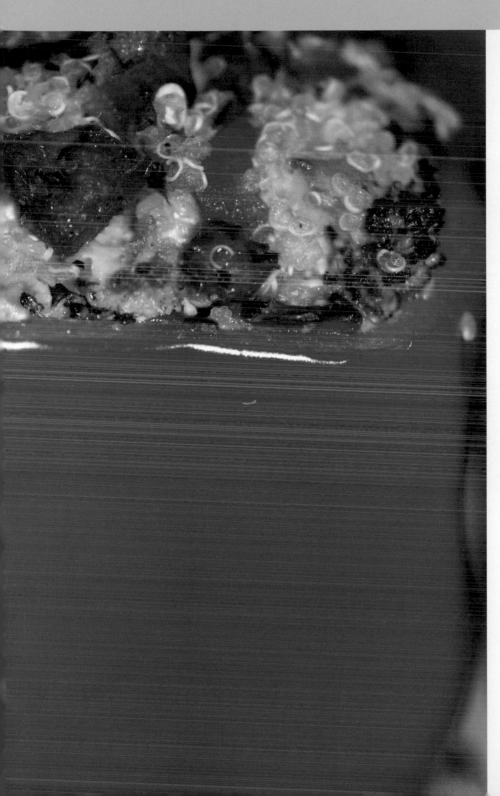

Vegetarians feel free to omit the chicken sausage here – you can either substitute soy "sausage" or just leave it out entirely.

Serves 4

1 cup quinoa
2 cups water, or chicken broth
4 medium bell peppers,
  varied colors
1 tablespoon olive oil
1 small onion, diced
1 clove garlic clove, minced
1 link organic chicken sausage (We like
  Applegate Farms)
¼ cup pine nuts
1 teaspoon ground cumin
½ small zucchini, diced
½ cup chopped spinach
½ cup chopped broccoli
1 tablespoon fresh oregano, chopped
¼ teaspoon sea salt, optional
2 ounces feta cheese, divided and crumbled

Per Serving:
290 Calories,
12g Fat (3g sat);
12g Protein;
36g Carbohydrate;
5g Dietary Fiber;
23mg Cholesterol;
340mg Sodium.

Sweet Potato Poblanos

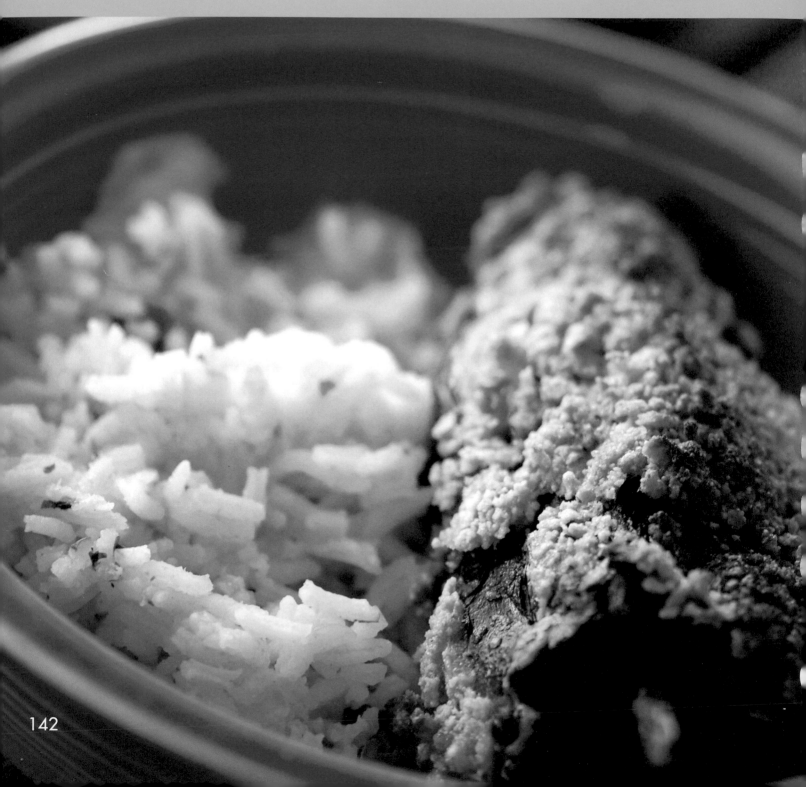

Bake sweet potatoes at 450°F for 45 minutes or until soft. Remove skin and mash until it is puréed. Combine sweet potato, cheese, pineapple juice concentrate, butter, salt and spices in bowl and set aside.

Poblanos: Make a small lengthwise slit on side of each chile. Carefully remove seeds with teaspoon (under running water). Arrange chiles on baking sheet. Place under broiler about 3 minutes or until they begin to blister and blacken. Rotate chiles and broil 3 minutes or until blackened all over. Place in a plastic bag to steam 5 minutes; remove skin.

Stuff chiles with about ¼ cup of the filling. Gently fold peppers closed.

Preheat oven to 350°F. Place flour, egg, and corn flakes in three separate shallow dishes. Dredge each pepper in flour, roll in egg, then coat with cornflakes. Heat oil in a large skillet over medium-high heat. Add peppers and cook until lightly browed all over, 4 to 6 minutes. Transfer to baking sheet lined with parchment. Bake peppers until cheese has melted and the filling is hot, about 20 minutes. Cool for 5 minutes and serve with plain yogurt or sour cream.

We completely covet these – the blend of sweet and spicy meets palate perfection. We've made them gluten-free. Poblanos are not overly spicy, but they do have a nice kick to them. They are loaded with vitamin C and relatively high in fiber.

Serves 4

4 large poblano chiles
1½ sweet potato
½ cup shredded Monterey jack cheese
1 tablespoon pineapple juice, frozen
*   concentrate, thawed*
2 teaspoons butter, melted
½ teaspoon salt
1 teaspoon cumin
¼ teaspoon oregano
¼ teaspoon nutmeg
¼ teaspoon cinnamon
½ cup rice flour
1 egg, slightly beaten
1 cup corn flakes, crushed
2 tablespoons canola oil

Per Serving:
331 Calories;
15g Fat (5g sat);
9g Protein;
42g Carbohydrate;
3g Dietary Fiber;
64mg Cholesterol;
462mg Sodium

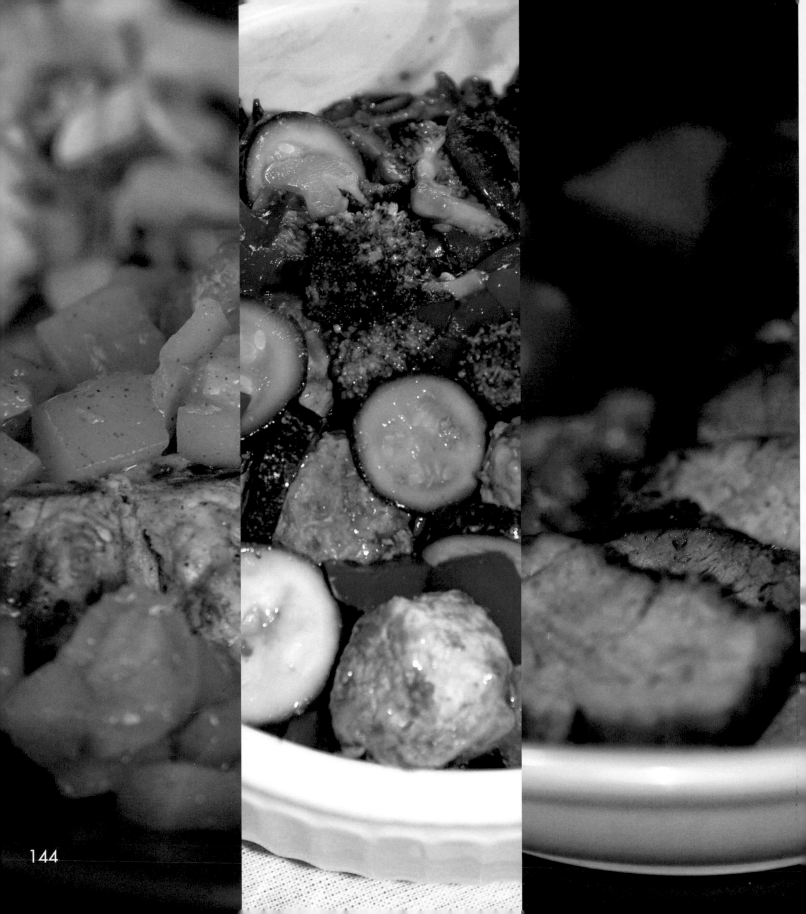

Red meat is not bad for you. Now blue-green meat,
that's bad for you! ~Tommy Smothers

Conscious Omnivore

Our love of food has taken us all over the map in terms of how we "define" ourselves dietarily. If we had to classify ourselves as any particular diet "type" we'd have to call ourselves conscious omnivores. We respect and honor all who choose their way of eating in a mindful and conscious way. We were vegan for many years, have dabbled in the raw movement and quite honestly love eating raw. Yet in our appreciation and celebration of many forms of food, there are times when we consciously choose to eat fish, poultry and on more rare occasions, meat and pork. We always choose free-range, organic meat and dairy products whenever possible. We feel this is not only the more humane way to go, but it is a healthier choice as well.

This pork has really great flavor and is quite easy to prepare. If you are pressed for time you can skip the brining and go straight for the smoky chipotle sauce and just grill away.

Serves 4

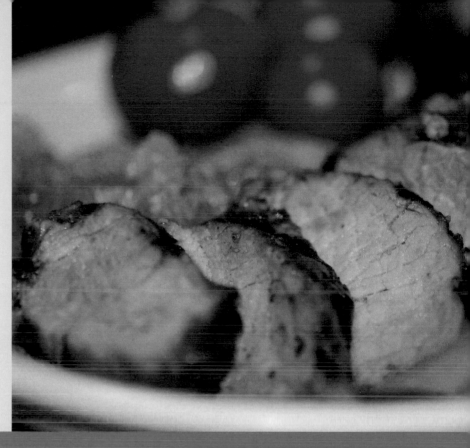

Fiesta Pork

1 pound pork tenderloin
2 cups water
1 tablespoon brown sugar
1 tablespoon sea salt
1 garlic clove
2 tablespoons chipotle chiles canned in adobo
1 cup barbecue sauce
2 tablespoons pineapple juice
2 tablespoons red onion, diced
2 tablespoons cilantro, chopped
1 tablespoon lime juice

Per Serving:
188 Calories;
6g Fat (2g sat);
22g Protein;
10g Carbohydrate;
1g Dietary Fiber;
51mg Cholesterol;
577mg Sodium.

Rinse pork with cold water and pat dry. In a large bowl or ziplock bag, combine pork with brown sugar, salt and garlic clove and cover with water so that salt and brown sugar dissolve. Refrigerate and marinate for an hour or more (up to about 4 hours).

Add chipotle chiles, barbecue sauce, pineapple juice, red onion, cilantro, and lime juice to food processor bowl fitted with steel blade. Pulse to purée until smooth. Cover and refrigerate until ready to use.

Remove pork from the liquid brine and pat dry once again. Brush liberally with chipotle barbecue sauce on both sides. Grill over medium heat until fully cooked, about 5 minutes on each side. Allow to cool a few minutes before slicing. Serve with Mango-Avocado Salsa (p. 248).

When we choose to eat red meat, we always go with free-range, grass-fed whenever possible. This meat is lower in saturated fat and higher in conjugated linoleic acid (CLA), which has anti-cancer and antioxidant properties. It's not only healthier for us, it's more humane for the animal.

Serves 4

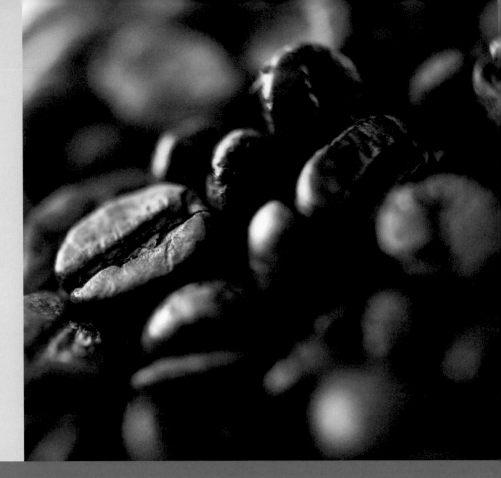

Java Steak

¾ cup strong brewed decaffeinated coffee
½ cup wheat-free tamari soy sauce
1½ tablespoons red wine vinegar
1 tablespoon gluten-free Worcestershire sauce (Lea & Perrins)
2 cloves garlic, minced

4 (4 to 6-ounce) beef fillets

Per Serving:
426 Calories;
32g Fat (13 g sat);
29g Protein;
4g Carbohydrate;
trace Dietary Fiber;
100mg Cholesterol;
450mg Sodium.

Combine coffee through garlic cloves in a large glass bowl and marinate the beef, covered, for at least 2 hours and up to 8 ours in the refridgerator. When ready to cook, preheat grill to medium high heat. Remove the steak from the marinade and grill for about 4 to 6 minutes on each side – until desired temperature and doneness is reached.

Serve over mixed salad greens drizzled with your favorite dressing or Divine Dressing (p. 82).

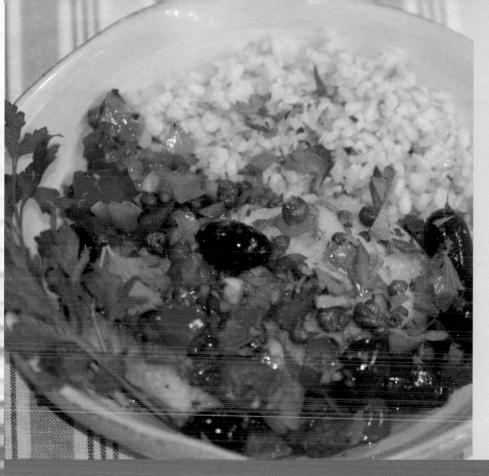

We typically cook pork in ways that we would cook chicken. The flavors of this dish are definitely Mediterranean with the olives and the capers, which we adore.

Serves 4

Mediterranean Pork Chops

Rinse and pat dry pork chops. Sprinkle lightly with salt and pepper and dust with rice flour. Heat 2 tablespoons of olive oil in a large skillet over medium high heat. Add pork chops and brown on each side (about 2 to 3 minutes each side). Remove pork chops from skillet and set aside temporarily.

Add onions and chopped garlic to the skillet and stir frequently for about 3 minutes. Stir in red wine, tomatoes, broth, vinegar, sugar and oregano. Bring to a boil and then lower to a simmer. Add pork chops back to the skillet as well as olives and capers and cover for another 5 minutes or until pork chops are cooked through to desired doneness.

Serve over noodles or rice with fresh chopped parsley on top.

4 (4 to 6-ounce) boneless pork loin chops
1 dash each of salt and pepper
2 tablespoons rice flour
2 tablespoons olive oil
1½ cups onions
2 cloves garlic cloves, chopped
½ cup dry red wine or Port
1½ cups Roma tomatoes, diced
1 cup low sodium chicken broth
¼ cup white wine vinegar
2 tablespoons turbinado sugar
2 teaspoons dried oregano
½ cup kalamata olives
2 tablespoons capers, drained and crushed
2 tablespoons chopped fresh parsley

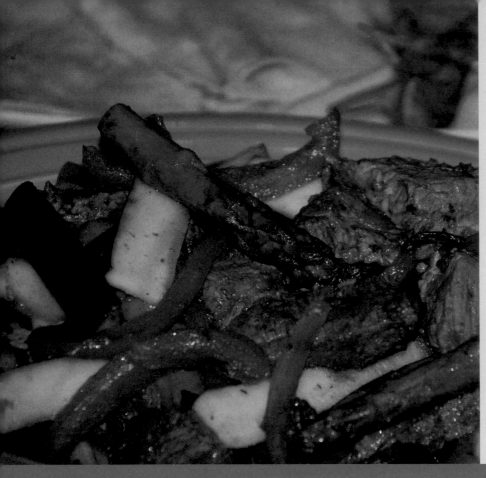

We recommend serving these on top of a bed of shredded lettuce with a little of Dakota's Ranch Dip, a side of salsa, guacamole, and some warm corn tortillas.

Serves 4

Per Serving:
267 Calories;
9g Fat (2g sat);
38g Protein;
8g Carbohydrate;
2g Dietary Fiber;
96mg Cholesterol;
243mg Sodium.

Naked Buffalo Fajitas

Thinly slice buffalo steak on the diagonal. Place buffalo in shallow bowl or dish and add salsa. Cover and refrigerate at least 30 minutes but no longer than 24 hours, turning buffalo occasionally.

Preheat cast iron skillet and add olive oil. Heat until medium hot, add red bell peppers and onion. Stir-fry until the onions are beginning to become translucent. Add the zucchini and asparagus spears and stir-fry until zucchini is slightly browned and beginning to get soft. Remove vegetables, add them to a bowl and keep warm.

Add buffalo slices to hot iron skillet and sauté or stir-fry until just barely cooked. You don't want to overcook buffalo. Add the vegetables to re-warm them completely and divide mixture onto 4 plates. Top with 1 tablespoon of guacamole.

1 pound buffalo sirloin steak, sliced thinly into ¼" strips
4 tablespoons salsa
1 tablespoon olive oil
1 red bell pepper
½ medium onion, sliced
1 medium zucchini, halved and sliced
¼ pound asparagus spears, chopped
4 tablespoons guacamole

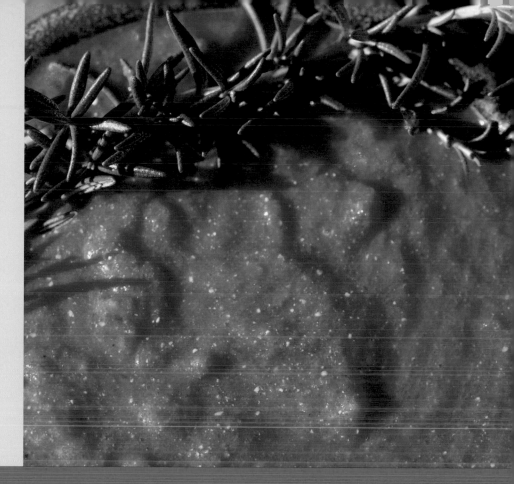

Rosemary has properties that may help boost the immune system, improve digestion and circulation and decrease inflammation in the body. Feel free to increase the amount of rosemary in the recipe if you are also a big fan.

Serves 4

Per Serving:
305 Calories;
21g Fat (5g sat);
23g Protein;
5g Carbohydrate;
1g Dietary Fiber;
62mg Cholesterol;
440mg Sodium.

Pagosa Pork Chops

¼ cup olive oil
3 cloves garlic, minced
1 tablespoon soy sauce
1 teaspoon chopped fresh rosemary
⅛ teaspoon pepper

4 boneless pork chops, 1-inch thick

Sauce
2 cups roasted red peppers
¼ cup feta cheese
¼ tablespoon garlic powder
1 dash fresh rosemary

For marinade, in a small bowl combine ¼ cup olive oil, garlic, soy sauce, rosemary, and pepper. Place pork chops in a 1 gallon self sealing plastic bag; pour marinade over chops, seal bag. Marinate in the refrigerator for 6-8 hours or overnight.

To prepare sauce combine red bell pepper, feta cheese, garlic powder and rosemary in a blender and blend until smooth. If needed, add a tablespoon of water. Place in a small pot, cover and heat over very low heat. Be careful that it doesn't boil. If it starts to simmer, remove from heat and keep covered. This will keep in the refrigerator for about 5 days.

To prepare the pork, first preheat the grill to medium-high. Remove the pork chops from the marinade. Place chops on the grill, decrease the heat to medium, and lower the grill hood and grill for 4-5 minutes. Turn chops and grill for 4-5 minutes more, until chops are just done. Serve chops with roasted red pepper sauce.

This is the perfect recipe when you have leftover chicken or roasted veggies. We like to use brown rice tortillas, which definitely taste a bit better when heated on a skillet. We often serve this with guacamole or a side of black beans.

Serves 4

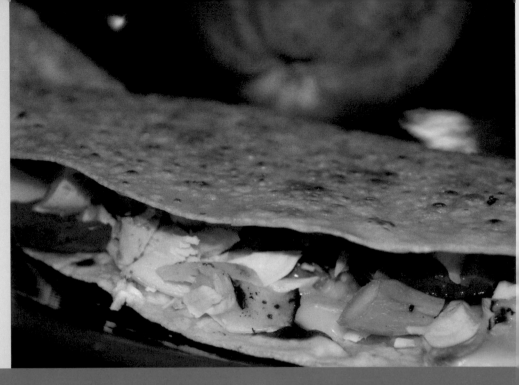

Mama Mia Quesadillas

8 asparagus spears
4 whole wheat or brown rice tortillas
½ cup diced red onions
¼ cup roasted red and yellow bell
   peppers, diced
½ cup marinated artichoke hearts, diced
8 ounces roasted chicken breast meat,
   shredded
4 ounces shredded lowfat cheddar cheese
Olive oil cooking spray
salsa - optional

Per Serving:
344 Calories;
11g Fat (3g sat);
30g Protein;
32g Carbohydrate;
4g Dietary Fiber;
54mg Cholesterol;
690mg Sodium.

Preheat oven to broil. Wash and trim asparagus spears. Place asparagus on a broiling pan lightly coated with cooking oil spray. Broil for about 2 minutes until asparagus has just started to brown. Remove from oven, allow to cool, and then chop asparagus into 1-inch segments and place in medium size bowl.

Add diced red onions, roasted bell peppers, artichoke hearts, and shredded chicken to bowl and mix together.

Coat a large nonstick skillet or griddle with cooking spray. Heat to medium high. Place 1 tortilla on the skillet at a time (or if you have room for 2 by all means make 2 at a time!). Spray the side of the tortilla that is not down with a very light coat of olive oil spray. Cook for about 1 minute and flip the tortilla over. Distribute about 1 ounce of shredded cheese and ½ cup of chicken and vegetable mixture onto one side of the tortilla. Fold the tortilla in half and turn the heat to low. Allow it to cook a few minutes and then flip the tortilla again. After you have successfully flipped, cook for another 3 minutes. Remove to cutting board and slice in half. Serve immediately.

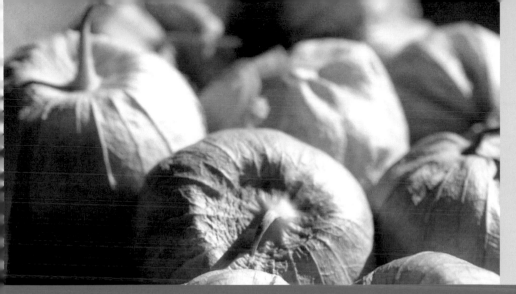

We have been making versions of these enchiladas for many years. Occasionally we will add black or pinto beans to the inside of the enchiladas, or just serve them with a side of beans – or our black bean salsa. When we are pressed for time or can't find good looking tomatillos then we use 505 Southwestern Green Chile salsa.

Serves 6

Bright Eyes Enchiladas

Remove husk from tomatillos, rinse and chop. Place in saucepan, cover with water and simmer until tender, about 5 to 7 minutes; drain and discard liquid.

Add tomatillos, garlic, jalapeno pepper, green chiles, cilantro, onion, tomatoes, honey, and salt to a food processor and purée.

Combine shredded chicken and spinach in a separate bowl and mix together until well blended. Add cumin, cayenne, salt, and pepper and mix again.

Soften tortillas either by frying on both sides in a small amount of vegetable oil and draining on paper towels, or by wrapping in foil and placing in hot oven until hot, or by placing in microwave in damp towel until heated. In the center of each warmed tortilla, place about 2 tablespoons of the chicken and spinach mixture and 1 tablespoon of the tomatillo mixture. Place filled enchiladas in greased 9×12-inch baking dish coated with cooking spray and pour remaining tomatillo sauce over the top. Sprinkle with cheese and top with green onions. Bake in a 350°F oven until heated through, and slightly browned on top, about 25 minutes.

1 pound fresh tomatillos
2 cloves garlic, peeled
1 jalapeño pepper, seeded and diced
1 cup diced green chiles
2 tablespoons cilantro leaves
2 tablespoons chopped onion
2 cups diced tomatoes, fresh or canned (no salt)
1 tablespoon honey
¼ teaspoon salt
2 cups cooked shredded chicken
1 package frozen cooked spinach, thawed and drained of excess moisture
½ teaspoon ground cumin
¼ teaspoon cayenne pepper
salt and pepper to taste
12 corn tortillas
1 cup shredded lowfat Jack cheese
½ cup green onion, diced

Per Serving:
348 Calories;
17g Fat (6g sat);
19g Protein;
33g Carbohydrate;
5g Dietary Fiber;
66mg Cholesterol;
323mg Sodium

153

Torrey's Peak Chicken

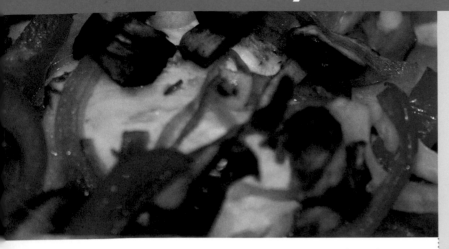

Fennel has impressive and unique phytonutrients that give it anti-inflammatory and antioxidant activity. In some studies these nutrients have even been shown to help prevent cancer.

Serves 6

2 ½ pounds boneless skinless
 chicken breast (each half cut into halves – this
 makes it easier to brown on each side and
 allows for more even cooking)
olive oil cooking spray
1 tablespoon olive oil
1 large red bell pepper, seeded and thinly sliced
1 large red onion, halved and thinly sliced
1 large fennel bulb, trimmed and thinly sliced
1 cup Portobello mushroom caps, chopped
3 cloves garlic, minced
1 tablespoon fresh rosemary
2 teaspoons orange zest
1 teaspoon fresh thyme
3 tablespoons red wine vinegar
½ cup dry white wine
¾ cup low sodium chicken broth, or vegetable broth
2 tablespoons tomato paste
sea salt, optional to taste

Heat a large skillet over medium high heat. Coat with cooking spray and add a tablespoon of olive oil. Arrange chicken breasts on the bottom of the pan and brown on each side (this should only take about 5 minutes).

Preheat oven to 350°F.

Transfer chicken to a large (9 x 13) baking dish and set aside.

While skillet is still warm, reduce heat to medium and add olive oil, bell pepper and onion. Stir-fry for about 4 minutes or so. Add the fennel and the mushrooms and stir-fry another few minutes. Add spices (garlic, thyme, rosemary, orange zest) and continue to stir over medium heat for another minute. Add the red wine vinegar, white wine, chicken broth, and tomato paste; stir until well mixed and bring the mixture to simmer for about a minute. Pour this mixture over the chicken and cover the baking dish with aluminum foil.

Bake for about 35 to 40 minutes. Let stand at least 5 minutes before serving. Serve with a side of greens and/or atop a small bed of whole grain pasta.

Per Serving
(divided by 6):
294 Calories; 5g Fat
(1g sat); 47g Protein;
11g Carbohydrate;
3g Dietary Fiber;
110mg Cholesterol;
255mg Sodium.

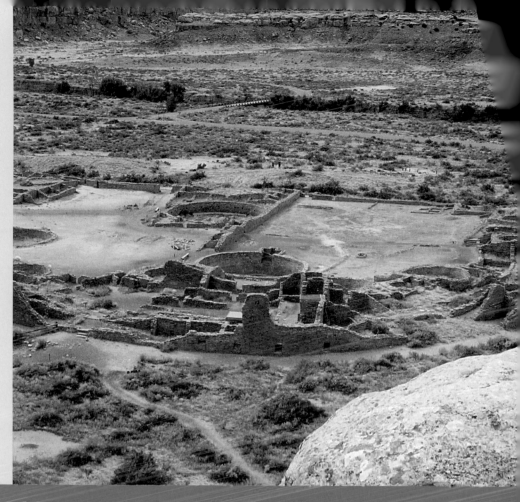

...n as a New Mexico-...ry, blending the awesomeness of the cocoa powder with the spice of the chile powder.

Serves 6

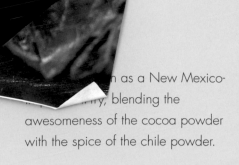

Per Serving:
328 Calories;
12g Fat (3g sat);
23g Protein; 33g
Carbohydrate;
4g Dietary Fiber;
58mg Cholesterol;
307mg Sodium.

Chaco Chicken

4 (6-ounce average) boneless skinless chicken breasts, diced
1 tablespoon olive oil
1½ cups diced onion
2 teaspoons ground cumin
1½ teaspoons chile powder
2 teaspoons cocoa powder
2 teaspoons ground cinnamon
3 15-ounce cans diced tomatoes
½ teaspoon sea salt
1½ teaspoons brown sugar

3 cups cooked basmati rice
2 limes, quartered for garnish
3 tablespoons fresh cilantro, chopped

Heat olive oil in 4-quart saucepan over medium-high heat. Sauté chicken and onion, stirring, until chicken is lightly browned. Add cumin, chili powder, cocoa and cinnamon and stir to totally coat the chicken. Add tomatoes, sea salt and brown sugar. Bring to a simmer and simmer for 8 to 10 minutes.

Serve over basmati rice and garnish with lime and cilantro. For an added treat offer a basket of M³ muffins (p. 41) to accompany the meal.

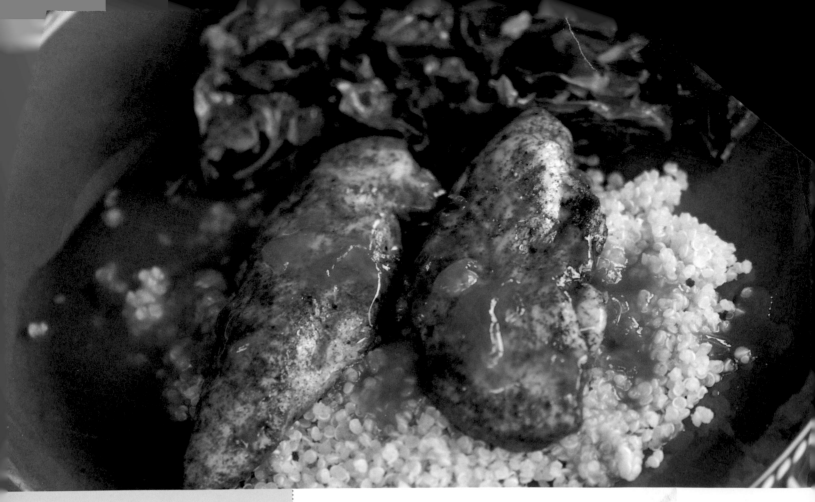

Serves 6

1 tablespoon olive oil
1 teaspoon ground cinnamon
½ teaspoon black pepper
½ teaspoon salt
1½ pounds chicken breast
tenderloins (**If tenderloins are not
available then use regular chicken
breasts sliced into halves or thirds)
⅔ cup apple juice
1 tablespoon arrowroot powder
1 tablespoon packed brown sugar
1 cup cherry preserves

Heat oven to 350°. Spray rectangular pan, 13 x 9 x 2 inches, with cooking spray. Mix oil, cinnamon, pepper and salt. Combine chicken and cinnamon mixture in a plastic ziptop and allow to marinate 30 minutes to 2 hours. Remove chicken from marinade and arrange in pan and bake uncovered about 25 minutes or until juice is no longer pink when centers of thickest pieces are cut.

While chicken is baking, mix apple juice, arrowroot powder and brown sugar. Mix juice mixture and cherry jam in saucepan. Heat to boiling, stirring constantly. Boil and stir 1 minute. Serve chicken over rice or quinoa; pour sauce over the top.

Per Serving:
288 Calories;
3g Fat (1g sat);
25g Protein; 41g
Carbohydrate;
1g Dietary Fiber;
61mg Cholesterol;
428mg Sodium

Cherry Chicken

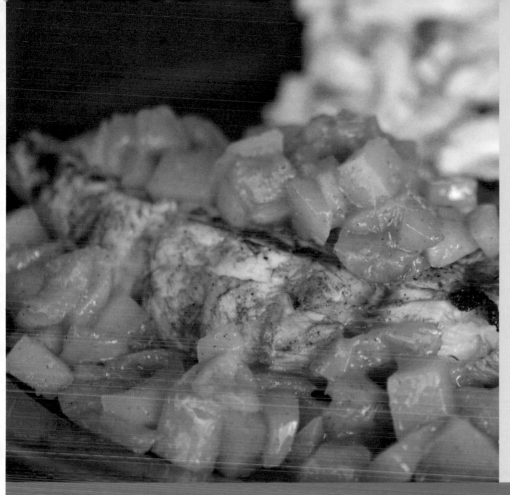

Mango is another fruit high in antioxidants like vitamin E, beta-carotene and selenium. Mango contains anticancer phenolic compounds and is a good source of iron.

Serves 6

Goldmine Chicken

Combine first 7 ingredients in a saucepan and bring to a boil. Reduce heat and simmer for 20 minutes, stirring occasionally.

In a ziptop plastic bag, combine the soy sauce, lime juice, curry powder and chicken. Marinate in refrigerator for 10 minutes, turning once. Heat grill over medium high heat. Grill chicken for about 5 minutes on each side or until fully cooked. Serve with mango relish and garnish with a lime wedge and Minted Cucumber Salad (p. 88).

Per Serving:
318 Calories;
3g Fat (1g sat);
43g Protein;
32g Carbohydrate;
3g Dietary Fiber;
99mg Cholesterol;
1456mg Sodium

Mango Relish:
2 cups mango, chopped and peeled
1 cup apple juice
⅓ cup dried apricot, diced
2 teaspoons cider vinegar
1 teaspoon fresh ginger, grated
¼ teaspoon allspice
⅛ teaspoon ground red pepper

Chicken:
⅓ cup tamari soy sauce
⅓ cup fresh lime juice
1 teaspoon curry powder
4 6-ounce skinless boneless chicken breast

157

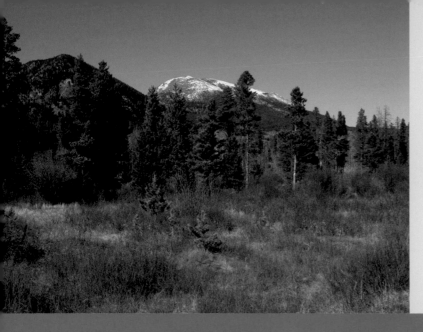

Fajitas are just plain fun – and when well garnished they can provide tons of vitamin C and healthy fat (think avocados!)

Serves 4

Frisco Fajitas

Cut chicken into thin strips. Add olive oil to a non-stick skillet and heat over high heat. Add garlic, onion, and peppers and sauté until almost tender - about 10 minutes. Add spices (chili powder through cayenne pepper) and continue to sauté another minute. Add chicken broth and bring to a low boil. Add chicken and stir until cooked through - about five minutes. Lower heat and cover to keep warm.

Wrap tortillas in aluminum foil and heat in oven for about 3 to 4 minutes or wrap in a clean dish-towel and heat in microwave for approximately 40 seconds.

Serve buffet style with optional garnishes set out in bowls so that each person can create their own fajita. Each person gets a plate with 2 warm tortillas (or 1 warm flour tortilla) topped with chicken fajita mixture and then fills the rest of his/her tortilla with optional toppings.

Per Serving:
356 Calories;
10g Fat (2g sat);
33g Protein;
34g Carbohydrate;
7g Dietary Fiber;
66mg Cholesterol;
239mg Sodium.

1 pound skinless boneless chicken breast halves
1 tablespoon olive oil
1 clove garlic, minced
1 medium onion, thinly sliced
1 medium red bell pepper, seeded and thinly sliced
1 medium green bell pepper, seeded and thinly sliced
¼ teaspoon chili powder
½ teaspoon oregano
¼ teaspoon cinnamon
¼ teaspoon cumin
¼ teaspoon thyme
¼ teaspoon cayenne pepper
½ cup low sodium chicken broth
8 corn or 4 whole wheat tortillas, warmed

Optional garnishes:
Salsa
Avocado (guacamole)
Shredded lettuce
Grated lowfat cheese
Lowfat sour cream

158

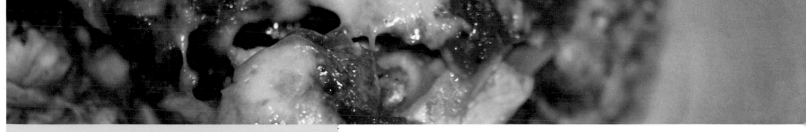

Lasagna is always a crowd pleaser. It is so satisfying and great for a dinner party or a chilly evening. You can make and bake two at the same time and freeze one for later or give the second one to a family in need. This is a great recipe to introduce tofu to your diet as an alternate source of protein. You can leave out the ground meat and go vegetarian, and you can use rice lasagna noodles to make this gluten-free.

Serves 16

15 lasagna noodles
½ cup part skim ricotta cheese
1 pound reduced fat, firm tofu (or cottage cheese)
1 egg, slightly beaten
1 large shallot, chopped
1 tablespoon olive oil
1 pound ground turkey or buffalo
4 cups marinara, divided
2 cups broccoli floret, chopped
2 small zucchini, chopped
2 cups spinach, chopped
¼ pound of fresh buffalo mozzarella cheese, sliced into small rounds
¾ cup lowfat mozzarella cheese, shredded
12 fresh basil leaves

Preheat oven to 375°F. Cook pasta according to directions, rinse with cold water and drain and lay flat on foil to cool. Alternatively, use no cook noodles (hint: most lasagna noodles can be used for the no pre-cook method).

In a small bowl combine ricotta cheese and tofu with egg, mashing and stirring with a fork until well combined (you can substitute cottage cheese for the tofu – or you can just use all ricotta).

In large nonstick skillet, sauté shallot in olive oil for about 5 minutes. Add ground turkey or buffalo and cook until meat is mostly cooked through. Add 3 cups marinara sauce to the meat mixture and add broccoli, zucchini and spinach and cook for about 5 more minutes.

Spread half-cup of plain marinara sauce in bottom of 13 x 9 x 2 pan. Arrange 4 noodles lengthwise over sauce and one across the bottom if needed to cover the pan, overlapping edges if necessary. Spread one-half of the ricotta-tofu mixture over pasta, followed by 1½ cups marinara-meat-veggie mixture. Repeat layers twice, ending with a third layer of pasta. Spoon remaining marinara sauce (and any remaining vegetables) over pasta. Top with fresh buffalo mozzarella and sprinkle with additional shredded mozzarella cheese, and fresh basil.

Cover lightly with foil – tented so that it won't stick to the cheese. Bake 30 minutes, remove foil and bake 10 more minutes or until hot and bubbly. Let stand 10 minutes before serving.

Per Serving:
470 Calories;
11g Fat (4g sat);
24g Protein;
68g Carbohydrate;
4g Dietary Fiber;
41mg Cholesterol;
349mg Sodium

Loaded Lasagna

Maple Roasted Turkey

When we introduced poultry into our diet and it and it was time to host our first family Thanksgiving, we were somewhat clueless as to how to prepare the big bird. The Vermonter in James surfaced, and maple syrup just came up naturally. With all the other traditional trimmings of the holiday, this big bird recipe fell right into place.

Serves 10-12

1 whole turkey (12 to 14 pounds), thawed, rinsed and patted dry inside and out (remove giblets and neck and reserve for making gravy stock or discard along with liver)
1 tablespoon butter, melted
2 tablespoons olive oil
2 tablespoons maple syrup
salt and pepper
1 pound shallots, peeled and halved
12 sprigs fresh thyme
3 cups water or (chicken or vegetable) broth to add to roasting pan
cooking oil spray
¼ cup maple syrup

Per serving
(based on 3-ounce
serving): 261 Calories;
11g Fat (3g Sat); 23g Protein;
16g Carbohydrate; trace
Dietary Fiber;
73mg Cholesterol;
79mg Sodium.

Position oven rack in lower third of oven and preheat to 350°F.

Set up a large roasting pan with a roasting rack that has been lightly sprayed with cooking oil spray. Place the turkey, breast-side up, on the rack in the roasting pan; pat dry with paper towels or clean kitchen towel.

Combine melted butter, oil, and maple syrup. With clean hands gently rub the mixture all over the turkey, including underneath the skin and onto the breast meat. Season generously with salt and pepper. Place thyme sprigs and shallot halves in the cavity. Close up the cavity by folding skin over and fastening with trussing needles or toothpicks. Tuck the wing tips under the turkey (bending them forward and securing underneath the neck cavity). Tie the legs together with kitchen twine. Add 3 cups of water (or chicken or veggie broth) to the roasting pan.

Loosely cover the turkey with aluminum foil and roast for one hour. After the first hour, baste the turkey with the pan juices/broth every 30 minutes until an instant read thermometer inserted into the thickest part of the thigh reads 125°F. This should take around 2 ½ hours, but be sure to check every half hour.

Increase the oven temperature to 400°F and continue roasting, but instead of basting, brush on a light coating of maple syrup every 15 minutes or so. Do this for about 45 minutes, or until the thigh temperature reaches 170°F. If the turkey breast starts to brown too quickly then go ahead and cover again (tenting) with aluminum foil that has been lightly sprayed with cooking oil spray. If pan juices begin to dry out, continue to add more water or broth, one cup at a time. When desired temperature is reached, transfer the turkey to a serving platter and again, cover with foil and allow to rest for at least 20 minutes.

Remove the twine and carve.

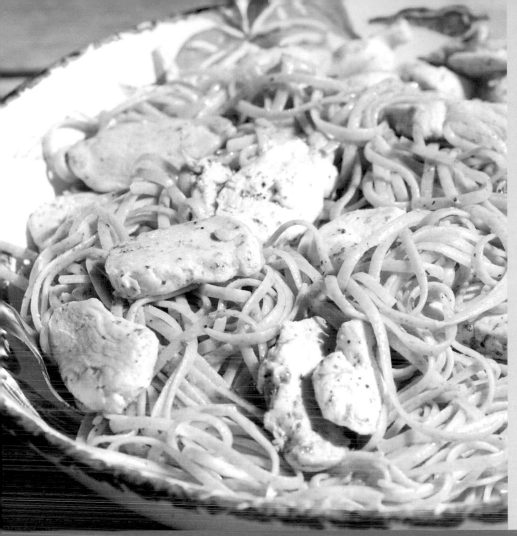

Pesto seems like an indulgence but truly the fat in pesto is generally coming from beneficial sources (minus the cheese). Pine nuts are high in protein and fiber, magnesium, and zinc. Olive oil is rich in monounsaturated fat, which may help prevent heart disease. Garlic may help protect the immune system and prevent heart disease. These are just a few reasons to love pesto!

Serves 4

Per Serving:
482 Calories;
24g Fat (4g sat);
22g Protein;
43g Carbohydrate;
2g Dietary Fiber;
40mg Cholesterol;
73mg Sodium

Pesto Pasta with Chicken

First prepare pesto: Place first seven ingredients in blender or food processor in the order listed. Cover and blend on medium speed, stopping occasionally to scrape sides, until almost smooth.

Cook and drain linguine as directed on package. While linguine is cooking, heat oil in 10-inch nonstick skillet over high heat. Add chicken and stir-fry until chicken is cooked through. Add about a teaspoon of pesto to the chicken to give it full flavor. Toss linguine with about 1 to 2 teaspoons pesto per serving. Add chicken and toss.

½ cup firmly packed fresh basil leaves
⅓ cup extra virgin olive oil
2 tablespoons pine nuts
2 tablespoons walnuts, or almonds
½ tablespoons fresh Parmesan cheese
1 clove garlic, or more as desired
salt and pepper, to taste

8 ounces uncooked linguine
1 tablespoon olive oil
1 pound free range chicken breasts
   cut in bite sized pieces

161

Perfect Pizza

We like to prepare the crust using a stand-up mixer or breadmaker (set on dough). It simplifies the kneading process tremendously. Warm the bowl of the mixer with warm water then add 1 cup warm water with yeast and whisk together lightly. Add olive oil, salt, and honey, stir briefly and allow to sit about 5 minutes. Add the all purpose flour and 1 cup of whole wheat flour to the yeast mixture. Then, attach the mixer bowl and the dough "hook" attachment to the mixture and mix on a low setting (we use setting #2) for about a minute. Add remaining ½ cup flour and mix until the dough comes away from the sides of the mixing bowl and sort of sticks around the dough hook. Remove dough from bowl and hook and then briefly knead dough on lightly floured surface until smooth and elastic, about a minute or so. Place in an oiled bowl, cover and let rise for 30 to 50 minutes.

Roll out dough to desired size and thickness. Sprinkle with cornmeal and brush with olive oil. Top with desired amount of marinara, tomato sauce or pizza sauce. Sprinkle evenly with different cheeses. Add toppings **

**We like to sauté onions until caramelized (in about a teaspoon of olive oil in a large nonstick skillet). We let the onions sauté about 5 minutes and then add the chopped bell pepper, sausage and mushrooms until they are all softened and slightly browned. We add spinach last until it is just wilted.

Preheat your oven and pizza baking stone at 425°F. Cook the pizza for about 13 to 18 minutes or until the crust is lightly browned.

**For the chicken sausage we like to remove the exterior casing and then slice or crumble the sausage and precook it prior to putting it on the pizza.

**Alternatively prepare our version of Gluten/Dairy-Free Pizza Crust (p. 242).

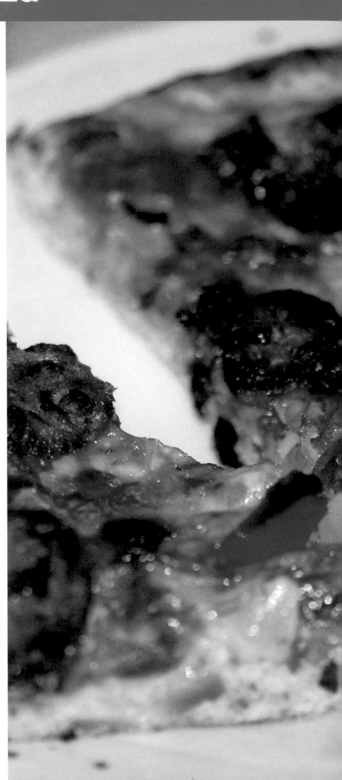

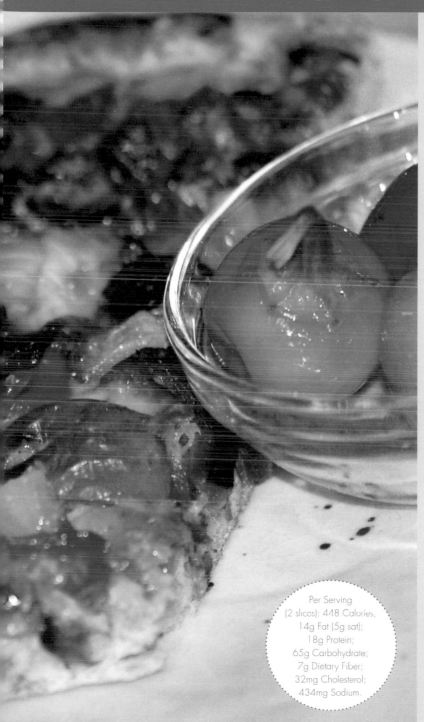

Pizza night is a given in the Rouse house. It is always
a weekend "event" and the kids will make their pizzas
of usually just cheese and the adults will pile on as
many vegetables as they can fit on one pie without
completely collapsing the crust. We usually make the
gluten-free version (see Basic Essentials) but admittedly
the crust below is easier to work with. We think pizza
has gotten a bad rap in terms of it's classification as less
than "health food." This pizza is loaded with vitamins
and minerals, fiber, lycopene and as long as you don't
eat the entire pie in one sitting, we believe it's a totally
balanced meal.

Serves 5

1 cup very warm water (110° to 120°F)
1 package active dry yeast (2¼ tsp)
½ teaspoon sea salt
1 tablespoon olive oil
1 teaspoon honey
1½ cups all-purpose flour
1½ cups whole wheat flour
1 teaspoon cornmeal

3 tablespoons marinara sauce
1 tablespoon olive oil
½ cup fontina cheese, shredded
½ cup mozzarella cheese
2 tablespoons Romano and/or Parmesan cheese
½ medium onion, thinly sliced
1 medium chicken sausage link, sliced**
½ medium red bell pepper, seeded and chopped
½ cup porcini mushroom, chopped
  (shiitake mushrooms also work great)
1 cup chopped baby spinach

Per Serving
(2 slices): 448 Calories,
14g Fat (5g sat);
18g Protein;
65g Carbohydrate;
7g Dietary Fiber;
32mg Cholesterol;
434mg Sodium.

163

If it seems like we use a lot of mushrooms, it's true, we do. We love them, especially shiitakes. Shiitakes are a symbol of longevity. They have a hearty and meaty texture and we love that they have potent effects on the immune system and may have a positive impact on heart health.

Serves 6

Per Serving:
217 Calories;
5g Fat (1g sat);
31g Protein;
9g Carbohydrate;
2g Dietary Fiber;
68mg Cholesterol;
353mg Sodium.

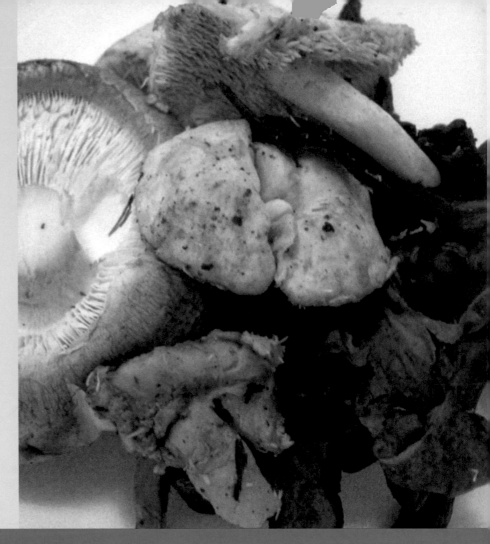

Shiitake Chicken

6 skinless boneless chicken breast halves
(about 1½ pounds)
1 tablespoon olive oil
¾ pound shiitake mushrooms, coarsely
chopped (5 cups)
1 medium leek, sliced (2 cups)
2 cloves garlic, finely chopped
2 tablespoons arrowroot powder
2 tablespoons water
2 cups chicken broth
½ cup dry white wine
1 teaspoon fresh oregano

Remove fat from chicken. Heat large nonstick skillet over medium heat. Add olive oil and chicken. Cook chicken in skillet about 12 minutes, turning once, until juice is no longer pink when centers of thickest pieces are cut. Remove chicken from skillet; keep warm.

Cook mushrooms, leek and garlic in same skillet about 3 minutes, stirring frequently, until leeks are tender. Mix arrowroot powder with water. Add arrowroot mixture, chicken broth, white wine, and oregano to mushroom mixture. Heat to boiling, stirring occasionally. Boil and stir about 1 minute or until slightly thickened. Add chicken; heat through. Serve over basmati rice or salad greens.

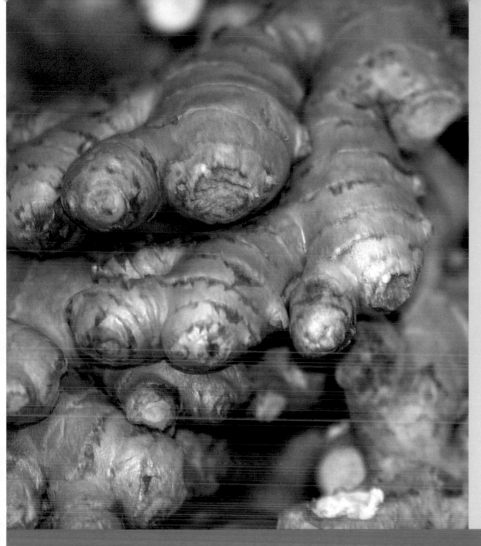

When you aren't cooking for a large gathering, sometimes it takes too much effort (and expense) to prepare an entire turkey. Turkey cutlets are a great way to go if you like turkey, but don't like the hassle of roasting an entire bird. We love the flavor combinations here.

Serves 4

Per Serving:
233 Calories;
8g Fat (1g sat);
25g Protein;
14g Carbohydrate;
trace Dietary Fiber;
64mg Cholesterol;
230mg Sodium

Spicy Ginger Turkey

Dust turkey with flour and sprinkle with salt and pepper. Remove excess flour by patting gently with (clean) hands. Heat oil in a large skillet over medium-high heat. Add turkey, brown on both sides until cooked, 3 to 4 minutes each side. Remove and keep warm.

Add ginger to the skillet. Cook 30 seconds, scraping up brown bits. Add brown sugar, red pepper flakes, and orange juice, stir to blend. Bring to a boil and cook, stirring occasionally, until slightly reduced, about 5 minutes. Return turkey and juices to pan. Simmer until warmed through and sauce thickens, about 3 minutes.

2 tablespoons all-purpose (or rice or potato) flour
dash of salt and pepper
3 teaspoons fresh ginger root, minced
2 tablespoons brown sugar
½ teaspoon red pepper flakes
1 cup orange juice
1 pound turkey breast cutlet
2 tablespoons olive oil
salt and pepper, to taste

165

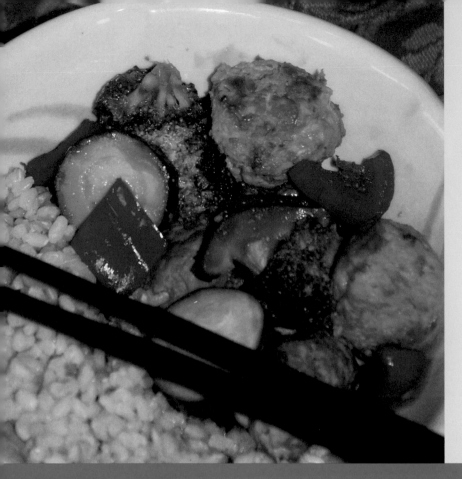

This is a relatively easy dish to prepare ahead of time by chopping all the vegetables and having them ready to go. The flavors all go really well together. We especially like this meal during the winter months.

Serves 6

Per Serving
(2 meatballs):
368 Calories; 5g Fat
(1g sat); 23g Protein;
68g Carbohydrate;
10g Dietary Fiber;
33mg Cholesterol;
579mg Sodium.

Mile High Meatballs

Mix turkey, bread crumbs and egg white. Divide mixture into 12 equal pieces; roll each piece into a ball. Lightly coat a 12-inch nonstick skillet with cooking oil spray. Heat the skillet over medium-high. Add meatballs to skillet and cook about 5 minutes, turning frequently to brown.

Add chicken broth, teriyaki sauce and vinegar to the skillet. Cover and simmer 10 minutes. Stir in mushrooms, bell pepper, broccoli, and zucchini. Cook 3 minutes, stirring occasionally, until bell pepper is crisp-tender and meatballs are no longer pink in center. Mix cornstarch and water; stir into sauce in skillet. Cook 1 to 2 minutes, stirring constantly, until thickened and bubbly. Serve over noodles or rice.

¾ pound ground turkey breast
¼ cup bread crumbs
1 egg white
1 cup low sodium chicken broth
¼ cup low sodium teriyaki sauce or tamari
1 tablespoon brown rice vinegar
2 cups shiitake mushroom, sliced
1 medium red bell pepper, cut into 1-inch
   pieces (1 cup)
1 large zucchini, cut into ¼-inch slices (2 cups)
1 cup broccoli florets, chopped
1 tablespoon cornstarch
2 tablespoons water

This is fettucine with an Asian flair. This meal is rich in tryptophan, anti-inflammatory nutrients and antioxidants and tons of flavor.

Serves 4

Per Serving:
483 Calories;
17g Fat (4g sat);
29g Protein;
8g Carbohydrate;
3g Dietary Fiber;
67mg Cholesterol;
166mg Sodium.

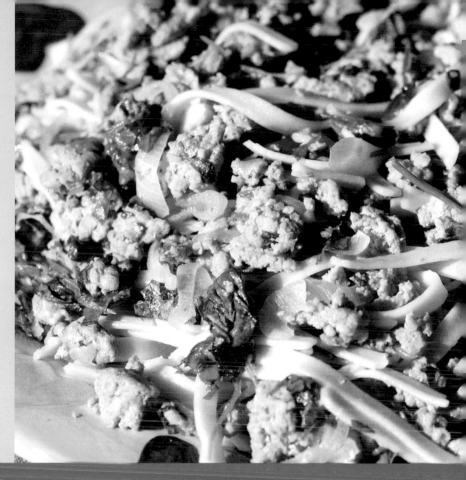

Urban Turkey

8 ounces brown rice fettucine (or Thai rice noodles)
2 tablespoons peanut oil
2 garlic cloves, minced
4 shallots, thinly sliced
1 tablespoon fresh ginger, sliced thin
½ teaspoon curry powder or paste
1 pound ground turkey breast
2 tablespoons fish sauce, available in Asian
   section of most grocery stores
½ cup low sodium chicken broth
½ teaspoon brown sugar
1 cup fresh basil
4 cups chopped baby spinach
salt and pepper, to taste

Cook the rice noodles according to directions on the package. Rice noodles vary considerably in texture and cooking times. Drain and set aside if they are finished cooking before the turkey.

Heat oil over medium-low heat in a large skillet. Add garlic, shallots, and ginger, stirring occasionally until the shallots are translucent, 2 to 3 minutes. Add the curry powder during the last minute. Turn the heat up to medium and add the ground turkey. Use a spatula to break up the clumps and cook until the turkey begins to turn whitish, about 4 minutes. Stir in fish sauce, chicken broth, and sugar. Bring to a simmer and add the basil and spinach. When the greens are wilted, gently mix the noodles into the skillet and cook for another minute or so. Season with salt and pepper if desired. Serve immediately while hot.

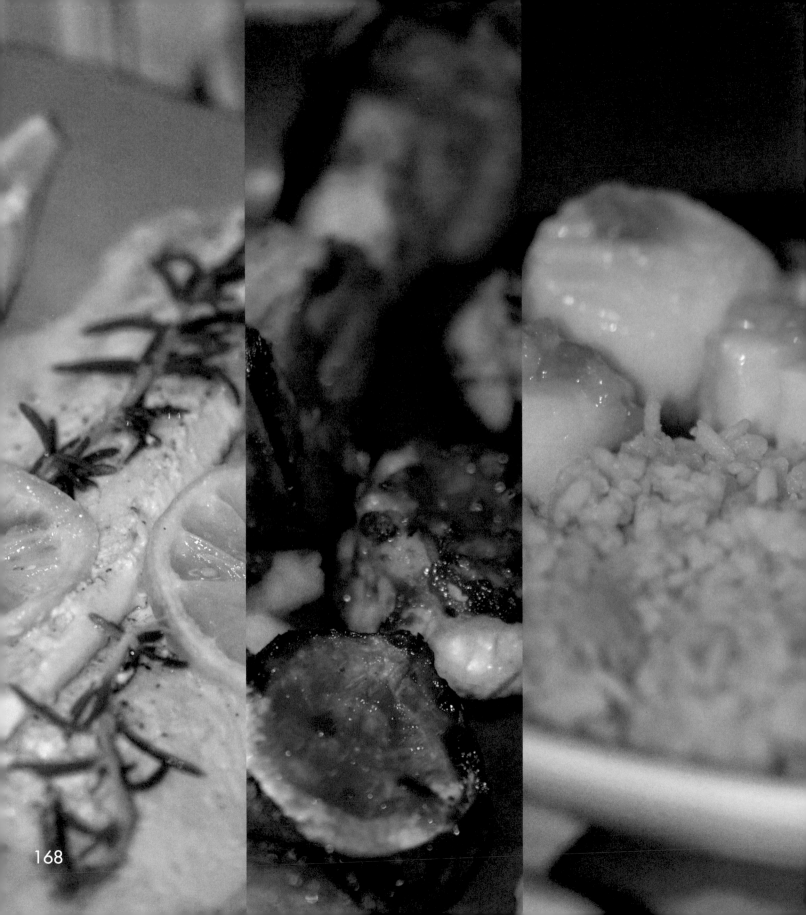

The spirit cannot endure the body when overfed, but, if underfed,
the body cannot endure the spirit. ~St Frances de Sales

Seafood Savvy

Nutrients in apricots, like beta-carotene, vitamin C, and fiber, may help protect the heart and eyes. Another positive effect on cardiovascular health comes from the scallops, which contain vitamin B12, omega-3 fatty acids, and magnesium. Citrus limonoids present in orange juice and lemon juice have been shown to help fight cancers of the mouth, skin, lung, breast, stomach and colon. Anti-inflammatory properties of ginger in addition to everything mentioned above make this one of our favorite scallop dishes.

Serves 5

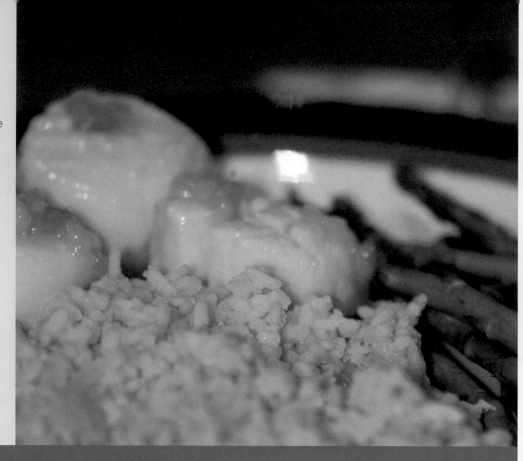

Western Slope Scallops

1½ pounds large sea scallops
2 tablespoons apricot preserves
1 tablespoon lemon juice
2 tablespoons orange juice
1 teaspoon fresh ginger root, peeled
  and finely minced
1 teaspoon olive oil

Rinse scallops and pat dry with paper towel or clean kitchen towel. Place scallops in glass baking dish. In a separate bowl, whisk together apricot preserves, lemon juice, orange juice, and ginger root and pour over scallops. Cover and refrigerate at least 30 minutes.

Heat olive oil over medium high heat. Add scallops plus preserve mixture and stir-fry until scallops are just cooked through. You can also skewer the scallops and grill or broil them.

Serve over brown rice, jasmine rice or whole grain pasta.

Per Serving:
151 Calories;
2g Fat (trace saturated);
23g Protein;
9g Carbohydrate;
trace Dietary Fiber;
45mg Cholesterol;
223mg Sodium.

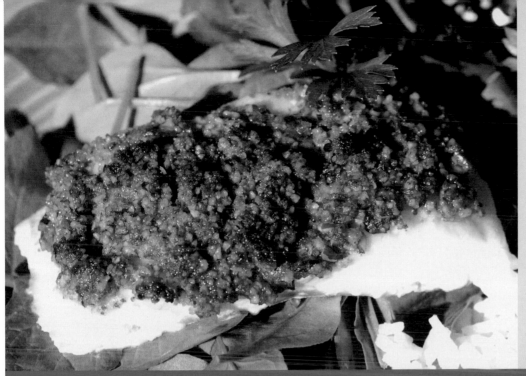

Our sister Tracy gave us a great salmon recipe, which we have adapted to halibut. Alaskan halibut is a real treat. Pacific halibut is still on the Environmental Defense Fund's "Eco-Best" list, so we're happy about that. Halibut supplies vitamins B6 and B12, a high amount of tryptophan, magnesium, and is a great source of omega-3 fatty acids.

Serves 4

Halibut in a Hurry

Preheat oven to 425°F. Line a baking dish or jellyroll pan with parchment paper or aluminum foil lightly coated with cooking oil spray.

In a food processor fitted with chopping blade, combine pecans, bread crumbs lemon zest, parsley, olive oil, salt and pepper. Process until the mixture is nice and crumbly.

Rinse the halibut fillets and pat dry, checking for any remaining bones and removing them gently. Note: we have a special pair of tweezers that we use just for removing fish bones - works great!

Spread a thin layer of mustard on the top of each fillet. On top of that spread ¼ of the nut crumble mixture evenly over the top of the fish.

Bake fish for about 15 to 18 minutes until it reaches desired "doneness." This is generally when the fish comes apart easily with a fork (like a flake). Serve with a lemon wedge or two. Great served with basmati rice and a side green vegetable like broccoli or asparagus.

½ cup pecans (or walnuts)
2 tablespoons bread crumbs
1 tablespoon lemon zest
1 tablespoon fresh parsley
2 teaspoons extra virgin olive oil
½ teaspoon sea salt
¼ teaspoon ground pepper
4 (4 to 6 ounce) halibut fillets
1 tablespoon Dijon mustard
lemon wedges, as garnish

Per Serving:
302 Calories;
15g Fat (2g Sat);
37g Protein;
3g Carbohydrate;
1g Dietary Fiber;
54mg Cholesterol;
375mg Sodium.

171

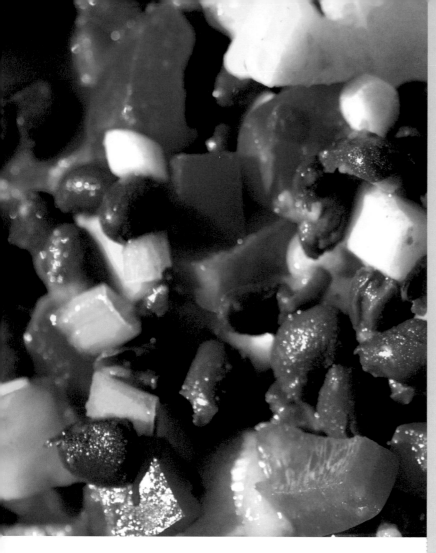

This recipe can serve as a wonderful appetizer or as a main course for about 4 people. Shrimp is a great protein source and this recipe could also be made with tofu. Curry and ginger offer wonderful anti-inflammatory properties. The black bean salsa adds a Caribbean flair in addition to heart-healthy fiber and vitamin C. Enjoy!

Serves 6

½ teaspoon grated orange peel
1 tablespoon orange juice
1 teaspoon curry powder
2 teaspoons lemon rind
¼ cup chopped fresh cilantro
1 tablespoon ginger, peeled and minced
1 pound raw medium shrimp, peeled and deveined

Black Bean Salsa
2 cups cooked black beans
1 medium mango, peeled and chopped (about 1 cup)
1 medium red bell pepper, chopped (about ½ cup)
⅓ cup sliced green onions (2 to 3 medium)
2 tablespoons orange juice
1 tablespoon rice wine vinegar
2 teaspoons lime juice

Combine first 6 ingredients in a sealable plastic bag. Add shrimp to bag and seal. Marinate in the refrigerator for at least 30 minutes. Meanwhile, prepare Black Bean Salsa by mixing all ingredients together. Then set aside in refrigerator.

Spray 10-inch nonstick skillet with nonstick cooking spray; heat over medium-high heat. Cook shrimp mixture in skillet, turning shrimp once, until pink. Divide salsa among 6 serving plates. Arrange shrimp on salsa.

Per Serving:
192 Calories;
2g Fat (trace sat);
21g Protein;
22g Carbohydrate;
6g Dietary Fiber;
115mg Cholesterol;
382mg Sodium.

Samba Shrimp

Our Favorite Salmon

Serves 4

Brine:
2 tablespoons brown sugar
1 tablespoon sea salt
3 cups water

1 pound salmon fillets
½ cup cherry preserves
¼ cup ketchup
2 chipotle chiles canned in adobo, with
  a little sauce
1 teaspoon thyme
1 tablespoon olive oil
Jalapeno-Lime Butter (p. 243)

Per Serving:
276 Calories;
7g Fat (1g sat);
24g Protein; 30g
Carbohydrate;
1g Dietary Fiber;
60mg Cholesterol;
320mg Sodium

Combine brown sugar, sea salt, and water in a heavy duty plastic bag or container with lid. Add salmon fillets, seal the bag, and place in refrigerator for 2 to 4 hours.

Meanwhile, combine cherry preserves through thyme in a blender and purée until smooth. Spiciness will depend on how many chiles you use. We usually use about 1½ plus a little extra adobo sauce. Drizzle in the olive oil and blend until just incorporated

Remove the salmon from the brine and blot dry with paper towels or a clean dish towel.

Preheat oven to broil.

Brush about a tablespoon of the chipotle-cherry sauce on top of the salmon. Place salmon on a broiler pan - we usually line it with aluminum foil to help with clean-up. We also find it easier to remove the skin when it cooks on the foil.

Broil salmon about 6 inches from the heat source for about 7 or 8 minutes until salmon flakes when tested with a fork.

Serve additional marinade on the side. We like to serve this salmon on top of brown basmati rice with a small teaspoon of Jalapeno-Lime Butter (p. 243).

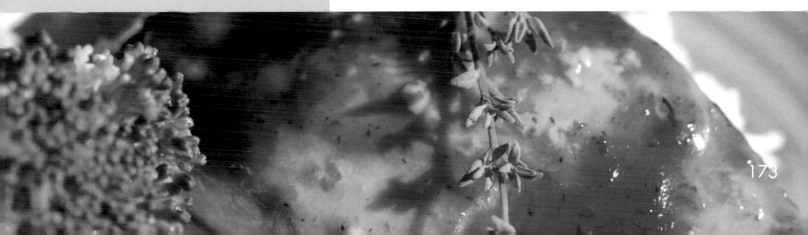

Radical Ratatouille

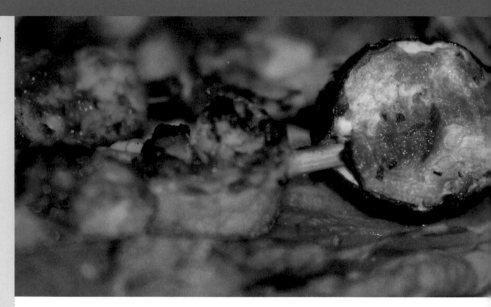

We've combined shrimp with one of our favorite summer dishes, ratatouille, and turned it into a kabob dish that is as easy as it is delicious. Shrimp and tofu add protein to make this a well-rounded dish for lunch or dinner. Tofu of course adds heart healthy phytonutrients. Both zucchini and eggplant add fiber, potassium, and great flavor, while onion adds quercetin and bell pepper adds vitamin C

Serves 4

1 pound medium shrimp, peeled and
*   deveined or 1 pound tofu, extra firm,*
*   cut in 1 inch cubes*
1 small eggplant (about ¾ of a pound),
*   cut in 1 inch chunks*
¾ teaspoon sea salt
olive oil spray
½ pound zucchini (2 small), cut in
*   1 inch chunks*
1 medium green bell pepper, cut in 1 inch
chunks
1 small onion, cut in 1inch chunks

Dressing:
2 tablespoons olive oil
¼ cup rice vinegar
2 tablespoons water
½ teaspoon sea salt
1 tablespoon fresh basil, chopped
1 clove garlic, minced
1 cup organic marinara or tomato sauce,
*   heated*

Rinse shrimp and set aside. Place eggplant in colander over bowl or sink. Sprinkle with salt. Let drain 30 minutes. Rinse and pat dry. Spray or brush olive oil onto grill rack. Heat coals or gas grill for direct heat.

Prepare dressing by blending or shaking olive oil, vinegar, water, sea salt, basil, garlic and tomato sauce.

Thread shrimp (or tofu), eggplant, zucchini, bell pepper and onion alternately on each of six 10-inch metal skewers, leaving space between each. Brush with dressing. (If you use wooden skewers be sure to soak them in water prior to threading on the food).

Place skewers across grill. Cover and grill kabobs 4 to 6 inches from medium heat 15 to 20 minutes, turning and brushing twice with dressing, until vegetables are crisp-tender and shrimp is cooked through.

Per Serving:
260 Calories;
12g Fat (2g sat);
28g Protein;
14g Carbohydrate;
5g Dietary Fiber;
138mg Cholesterol;
616mg Sodium

174

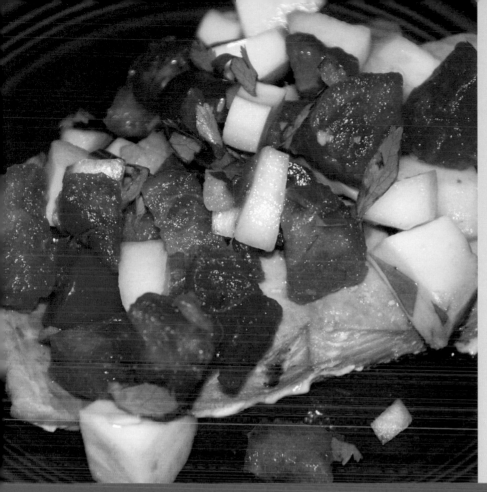

This is the perfect meal for an outdoor summer night. Be sure to choose wild salmon. Wild salmon is rich in essential omega-3 fatty acids, tryptophan, protein, vitamins B6, B12, niacin, selenium, and magnesium.

Serves 4

Per Serving:
356 Calories;
16g Fat (3g sat);
37g Protein;
17g Carbohydrate;
3g Dietary Fiber;
88mg Cholesterol;
262mg Sodium.

Summertime Salmon

Rinse salmon and pat it dry. Brush lightly with olive oil and squeeze fresh lime juice over top of filets. Sprinkle with a dash of salt and pepper if desired. Refrigerate for at least 15 minutes or until ready to grill. Grill salmon over medium high heat until you reached desired doneness.

To prepare salsa, combine all ingredients in a medium size bowl and toss. Refrigerate for at least 30 minutes prior to serving. Serve generously on top of salmon.

4 salmon fillets
2 teaspoons olive oil
2 tablespoons fresh lime juice
1 dash salt
1 dash pepper

Salsa:
1 medium cucumber, peeled, seeded and diced
½ cup red onion, diced
¼ cup cilantro, chopped
2 cups watermelon, seeded and cubed in ½ inch pieces
½ cup chopped tomatoes
1 medium avocado, cubed
4 tablespoons fresh lime juice

Just for the Halibut Tacos

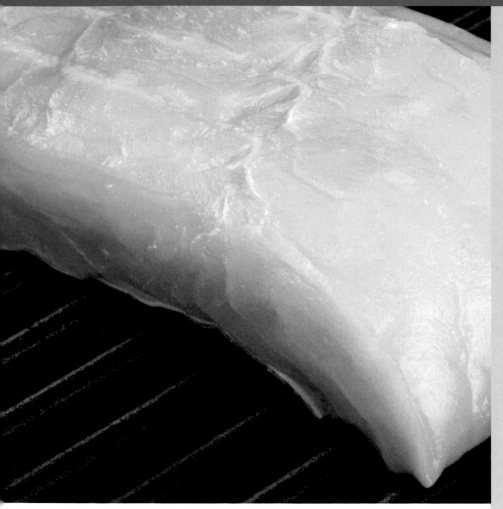

After a trip to Sayulita, Mexico we fell in love with fish tacos. This recipe is a healthier version of them.

Serves 4

2 tablespoons lime juice
1 teaspoon olive oil
1 pound Alaskan halibut fillets, about 1 inch thick
8 corn tortillas (6 to 8 inches in diameter), warmed
1 cup cabbage, shredded
1 small red bell pepper, chopped (½ cup)
1 medium onion, chopped (½ cup)
1 medium avocado, diced

⅓ cup lowfat mayonnaise
1 cup nonfat yogurt
½ teaspoon chili powder
1 tablespoon ketchup
¼ teaspoon ground cumin
1 dash hot sauce
juice from one lime

Mix lime juice and oil; brush over fish. Preheat grill to medium-high. Grill fish 10 to 15 minutes, turning once, until fish is cooked through and flakes easily. We find it easiest to place fish on a piece of aluminum foil to prevent it sticking to the grill.

Break fish into large flakes, or cut into 1-inch pieces. Spoon scant ½ cup fish onto center of each tortilla. Top with cabbage, bell pepper, onion, and avocado. Serve with white sauce. For the white sauce, combine mayonnaise through juice of lime in a small bowl.

Per Serving:
466 Calories;
21g Fat (3g sat);
31g Protein; 39g Carbohydrate;
6g Dietary Fiber;
46mg Cholesterol;
337mg Sodium.

176

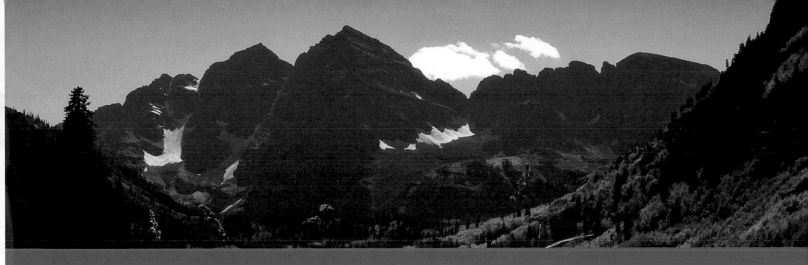

Maroon Bells Mahi

In one four week long clinical trial published in the Journal of Nutrition, individuals who ate a serving of pistachios daily improved their risk factors for heart disease without gaining weight. So for those who are "nut phobic" because you fear the fat content, it is time to let go of outdated thinking. We're talking good fat, healthy fat – good for the brain, mood, libido, hormonal balance, and let's face it, good for the soul.

Serves 4

½ cup pistachio nuts, shelled
¾ cup basil leaves, packed
2 teaspoons fresh garlic, minced
2 tablespoons olive oil
2 tablespoons Romano cheese, shredded
¼ teaspoon fresh ground pepper
4 (4 to 6 ounce) mahi mahi or halibut fillets
olive oil spray
salt and pepper, to taste
1 small lemon, as garnish

To prepare pesto, combine pistachio nuts through fresh ground pepper in a food processor fitted with blade attachment. Process on low until well mixed and nearly puréed.

You can either prepare the fish on the grill, in the oven or stovetop. If you prefer to grill it , then preheat your grill to medium high. Oven preheat to 400°F. Lightly coat fillets with olive oil spray. If you prefer the stovetop method, then add two teaspoons of olive oil to a heavy large skillet and heat over medium-high heat. The next step is the same for all methods: lightly sprinkle fish with salt and pepper if desired.

Place fish on grill and grill until just cooked through (about 4 minutes each side). Spread pesto on top of fish after you have flipped it one time. If using a skillet, saute' until lightly browned on each side and cooked through (about 4 to 5 minutes each side). Again, spread pesto after you have flipped the fish once. If baking, place in large baking dish coating with cooking spray, spread about a tablespoon of the pesto on top of each fillet and bake for 15 minutes or until fish flakes and is cooked through.

Serve atop greens or rice (or both!). Garnish with a generous slice of lemon.

Per Serving:
270 Calories;
16g Fat (3g sat);
26g Protein;
6g Carbohydrate;
2g Dietary Fiber;
86mg Cholesterol;
144mg Sodium.

Debra learned to fish when she lived in Idaho during high school. She caught mostly rainbow trout in those days and the only way she liked to cook it was by wrapping it in foil and grilling or baking it. Here is a modified version of that recipe. It also works nice to add a few slices of zucchini on the fish or to experiment with different varieties of trout. Antioxidant-rich rosemary really makes this dish wonderful and for those fans of the Mediterranean lifestyle, this one is perfect for you!

Serves 5

Per Serving:
374 Calories;
23g Fat (4g sat);
38g Protein;
5g Carbohydrate;
trace Dietary Fiber;
105mg Cholesterol;
309mg Sodium.

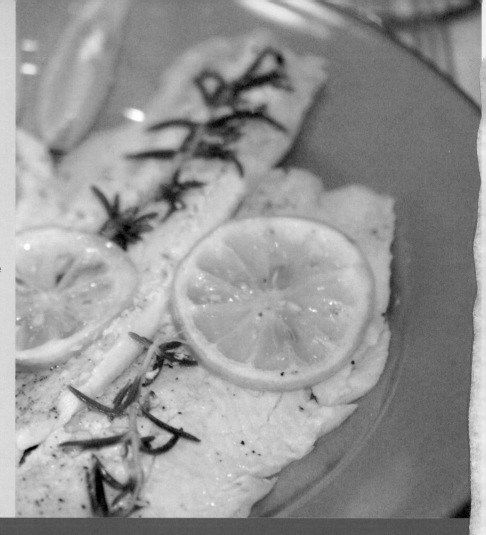

Rosemary Trout

4 (½ pound) trout fillets (red ruby
   trout is wonderful if you can find it)
½ teaspoon salt, divided
¼ teaspoon pepper
4 sprigs rosemary (each about 3 inches long)
8 thin slices lemon
4 teaspoons olive oil
4 to 8 lemon wedges for garnish
Aluminum foil (if using the grill method)

Preheat grill to medium or preheat oven to 350°F. Sprinkle fish with salt and pepper. Place 1 sprig rosemary and 2 slices lemon on top of each fish. Drizzle one teaspoon olive oil over each filet. Wrap fish in aluminum foil coated with cooking spray or place in oven-safe glass pan coated lightly with cooking spray.

Grill fish about 15 to 20 minutes, turning once, until fish flakes easily with fork (or bake for 15 to 20 minutes and brush with oil halfway though).

To serve, slide trout off of skin and onto serving plate. Garnish with fresh rosemary and lemon wedges. Excellent with steamed vegetables and rice.

Santa Fe Shrimp

Peel shrimp. (If shrimp are frozen, do not thaw; peel in cold water.) Make a shallow cut lengthwise down back of each shrimp; wash out vein.

Heat oven to 250°F. Wrap tortillas in aluminum foil, or place on heatproof serving plate and cover with aluminum foil. Heat in oven about 15 minutes or until warm. Another option would be to cook in a small amount of oil on the stovetop.

Heat oil in 10-inch skillet over medium heat. Cook shrimp, peppers and onion in oil. Sprinkle with garlic powder and black pepper (Note: You can also grill these on the barbeque over medium high heat - best on a skewer)

Heat beans in microwave-safe dish or on the stove top and then divide evenly among tortillas (about ¼ cup per tortilla). Follow with ¼ shrimp/pepper mixture. Top with salsa (see directions below).

For the salsa, combine all the ingredients and toss lightly to mix.

*we use gluten-free brown-rice tortillas – you can also substitute 2 corn tortillas for each flour tortilla.

As you may notice from many of our recipes, we have a special fondness for the flavors of Mexico. This is a fajita-like recipe. Shrimp cook up quickly which makes this a nice choice when you are pressed for time – especially when pre-sliced bell peppers and onions are also fairly easy to come by in most grocery stores. The salsa is more time consuming, but always worth it. The only thing differentiating this salsa from others is the yellow tomato. Buy them at their peak during the summer months – or make the salsa from heirloom tomatoes, which are amazing.

Serves 4

1 pound large shrimp, uncooked
1 red bell pepper, stem and seeds removed and sliced thin
1 green bell pepper, stem and seeds removed and sliced thin
1 yellow bell pepper, stem and seeds removed and sliced thin
½ medium onion, sliced
½ teaspoon garlic powder
¼ teaspoon black pepper
4 flour tortillas (7 or 8 inches in diameter)*
1 cup pinto beans, refried, low salt

Homemade Salsa
1 large tomato, diced
1 large avocado, diced
1 tablespoon lime juice
1 large yellow tomato, diced
½ medium onion, diced
¼ teaspoon sea salt
½ small jalapeno chile pepper, diced
Garnish with fresh cilantro

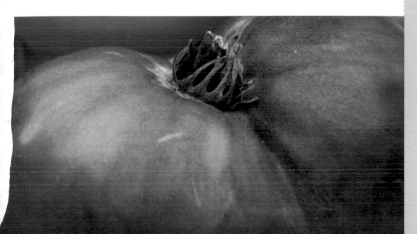

Per Serving:
393 Calories;
13g Fat (2g sat);
30g Protein; 43g
Carbohydrate;
6g Dietary Fiber;
173mg Cholesterol;
688mg Sodium.

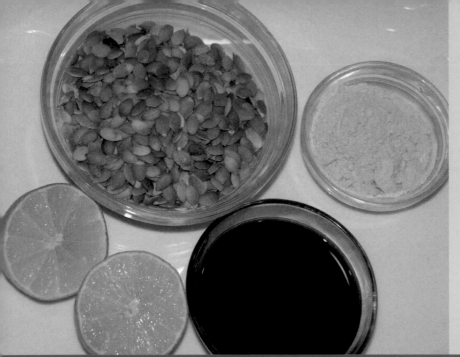

Inspired by our sister Tamara's stand-by recipe of baked salmon with a crust made from wasabi peas, we adapted our recipe to create a gluten-free version. Wasabi, Wasabia japonica, is related to watercress, but most Westerners are familiar with Japanese horseradish, which is easier to find in supermarkets and less expensive than authentic wasabi. For this recipe, Japanese horseradish powder will work just fine. We love the fiery kick combined with the freshness of the lime.

Serves 4

Wildfire Salmon

Preheat oven to 425°F. In a medium bowl, whisk together 1 tablespoon of wasabi powder with tamari, egg yolk, and olive oil.

Combine 1 tablespoon wasabi powder, lime zest, lime juice, bread crumbs, ground pumpkin seeds, and coarse salt. Cover rimmed baking sheet with parchment or with aluminum foil lightly coated with cooking spray. Arrange salmon fillets, skin side down, on prepared baking sheet.

Spread a layer of the wasabi soy sauce mixture on top of each fillet. Press about 1 tablespoon of the wasabi-lime-breadcrumb mixture on top of that, covering tops completely.

Bake for 15 minutes until salmon is cooked through and tops are lightly browned.

Serve salmon with warm brown or basmati rice and a side of steamed or sautéed kale.

2 tablespoons tablespoon wasabi powder, divided
1 tablespoon wheat-free tamari soy sauce
1 egg yolk
1 tablespoon olive oil
1 tablespoon fresh lime zest
2 tablespoons fresh lime juice
4 tablespoons bread crumbs (we prefer to make our own from gluten free bread)
2 tablespoons ground pumpkin seeds
¼ teaspoon coarse salt
4 (6-ounce) salmon fillets
Lime wedges

Per Serving:
286 Calories;
11g Fat (2g sat);
36g Protein;
8g Carbohydrate;
1g Dietary Fiber;
142mg Cholesterol;
543mg Sodium.

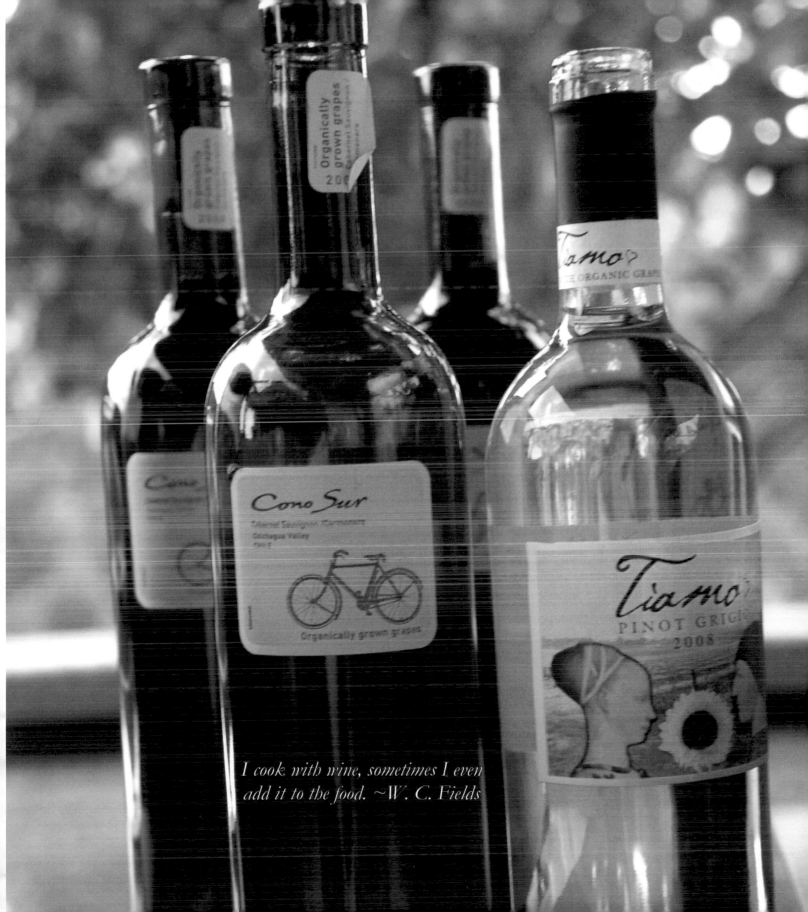

I cook with wine, sometimes I even add it to the food. ~W. C. Fields

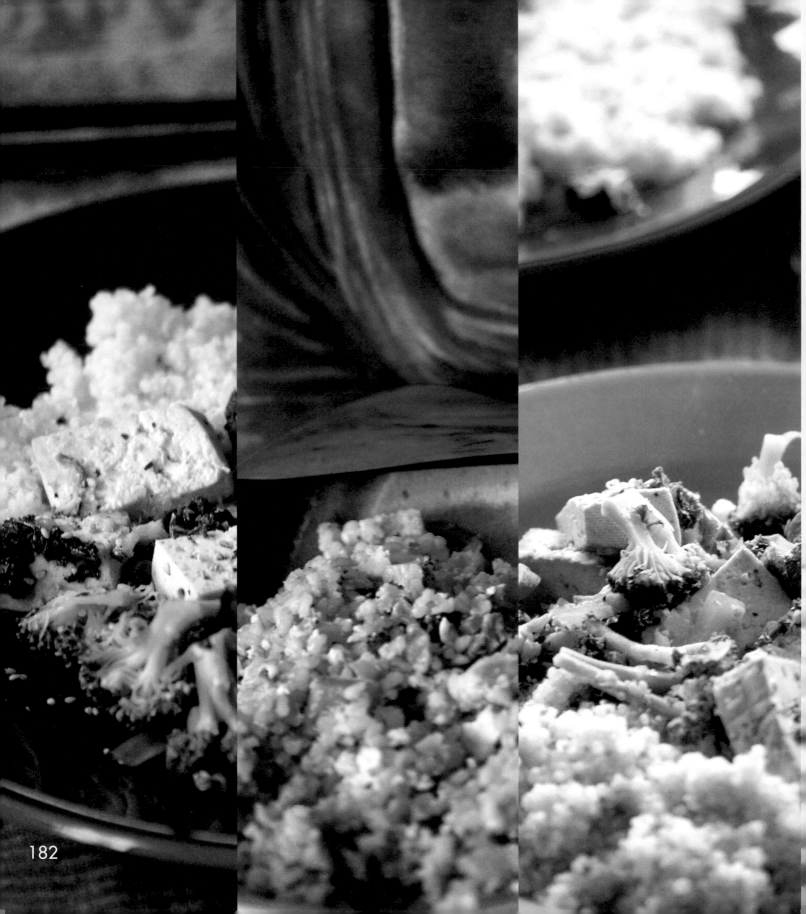

Cooking is like love. It should be entered into with abandon or not at all.
~Harriet Van Horne

Vegetarian

These are not the only vegetarian recipes in the cookbook, but they all make a great main course so we decided to give them their own section. People choose a vegetarian lifestyle for many reasons — health, environment and/or ethical reasons. We encourage you to take a look at your own biochemical individuality and see what works best for you.

This is a substantially filling meal in itself, full of fiber and antioxidant goodness. Pumpkin seeds have been studied for their potential prostate benefits.

Serves 6

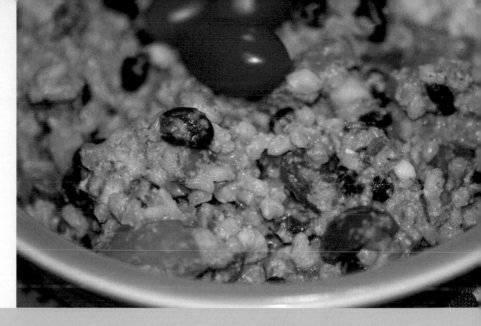

Mesa Verde Medley

¾ cup shelled pumpkin seeds
1 teaspoon olive oil
12 green onions, chopped (about 1 cup)
3 cloves garlic, minced
2 cups romaine lettuce, chopped
1½ cups low sodium vegetable broth
1 cup cilantro, chopped
2 tablespoons lime juice

2 cups cooked brown rice
1 cup black beans
1 cup red bell pepper, chopped
1 cup yellow bell pepper, chopped
1 medium avocado, chopped
1 cup cherry or grape tomatoes

Per Serving:
336 Calories;
9g Fat (1g Sat);
16g Protein;
53g Carbohydrate;
11g Dietary Fiber;
0mg Cholesterol;
156mg Sodium.

To make sauce: Toast pumpkin seeds 3 to 5 minutes in skillet over medium heat, stirring or shaking pan often.

Add oil to pumpkin seeds in skillet. Add green onions and garlic and sauté 2 minutes, or until soft.

Purée lettuce, broth, cilantro, and ½ cup pumpkin seed/green onion mixture in food processor or blender until smooth. Transfer back to skillet with remaining seed mixture, and simmer 15 minutes over medium heat.** Stir in lime juice and season to taste with pepper and a dash of sea salt.

Combine rice, beans, bell pepper and avocado in a large bowl and toss to combine. Add pumpkin seed sauce and toss lightly until the sauce is well mixed with the salad. Top with grape or cherry tomatoes.

**You may choose to purée more or less of the pumpkin seed mixture with the lettuce, broth and cilantro — this will alter the overall consistency of the sauce and the crunchiness that you desire in the salad. For additional crunch you may choose to add additional toasted pumpkin seeds on top.

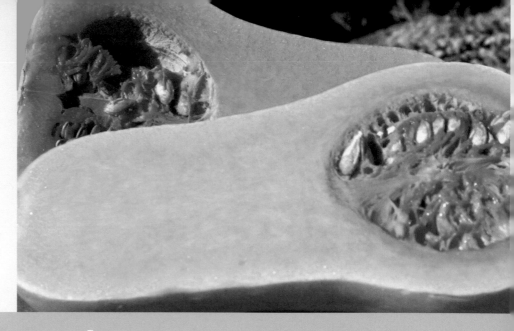

Yummy yummy!! This is a super creamy and scrumptious dish – we'll sometimes serve it as a side and other times it is the main attraction. You can vary the level of indulgence by the amount of cream you use. Here we use part milk, part half and half, but feel free to experiment.

Serves 6

Powered Up Pasta

1 pound whole wheat or gluten-free penne pasta
1 tablespoon olive oil
2 garlic cloves, chopped
1 medium shallot, chopped
1 small butternut squash, peeled, seeded, and cubed
1 cup low sodium vegetable broth
½ cup lowfat 2% milk
½ cup half and half
¼ cup Parmesan cheese
salt and pepper
Optional spices: nutmeg, thyme, or rosemary work great in this dish – add about ¼ teaspoon when stirring in the milk and cheese.

Per Serving:
474 Calories;
7g Fat (3g sat);
19g Protein;
93g Carbohydrate;
12g Dietary Fiber;
12mg Cholesterol;
184mg Sodium.

Place a large pot of water on the stove and bring to a boil. While waiting for the water to boil, add olive oil to a large skillet and place over medium-high heat. Add garlic and shallots to olive oil and stir until fragrant, about 1 minute. Add butternut squash and continue to cook and stir about 3 or 4 minutes. Add vegetable broth to this mixture, cover and reduce heat to low, about 15 minutes.

When the water is boiling, add pasta and cook until done - al dente preferably. Note: if the pasta takes less than 15 minutes to cook you may want to start cooking it after your sauce is made.

When the butternut squash is fork tender, remove from heat. Allow the mixture to cool slightly then purée in a blender or food processor. While blending, add milk, half and half, and cheese. Blend until smooth.

When pasta is ready, drain all of the water off by pouring everything into a strainer or colander. Then return the pasta to the pot and add butternut squash mixture. Stir in until everything is wonderfully coated and creamy.

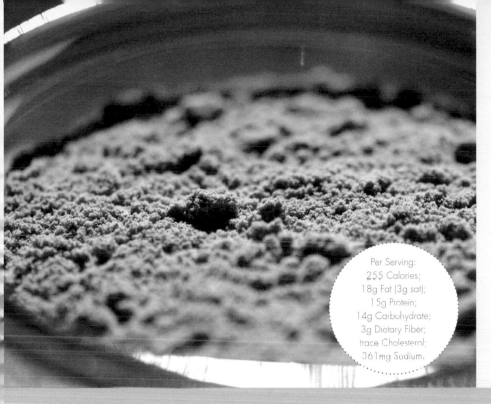

Per Serving:
255 Calories;
18g Fat (3g sat);
15g Protein;
14g Carbohydrate;
3g Dietary Fiber;
trace Cholesterol;
361mg Sodium.

We constantly sing the praises of curry for it's anti-inflammatory benefits, but coconut milk has some impressive qualities as well. Coconut milk contains fat in the form of medium-chain triglycerides (MCTs) that may actually assist with weight loss. Coconut milk is also rich in antioxidants that nurture the skin, hair, and vision, and lauric acid, that has antiviral and antibacterial properties.

Serves 4

Coconut Curry Tofu

In a large wok or sauté pan, heat 1 teaspoon olive oil over medium high heat. Add tofu and soy sauce and stir-fry about two minutes. Flip tofu so that a different side is in contact with your pan and stir-fry another two minutes until tofu just starts to brown. Flip tofu again, cook a few more minutes and then remove from pan and set aside temporarily.

In the same wok or pan, add another teaspoon of olive oil and heat over medium high. Add broccoli and red bell pepper and stir-fry about 3 minutes and then remove from heat.

In a medium size bowl or two-cup capacity glass measuring cup, whisk together coconut milk through basil leaves until well combined. Add tofu to broccoli and red bell pepper mixture and stir in the coconut curry basil mixture. Turn heat back on to medium and cook about 3 more minutes. Garnish with slivered almonds.

This mixture is delightful served atop jasmine rice or rice noodles.

15 ounces firm tofu, drained and cubed
1 tablespoon low sodium soy sauce
2 teaspoons olive oil, divided
1 cup broccoli florets
1 medium red bell pepper, seeded and chopped
¾ cup light coconut milk
¼ cup low sodium vegetable broth
1 tablespoon low sodium soy sauce
1 tablespoon fresh lemon juice
1 teaspoon minced fresh ginger
1 teaspoon curry powder
2 teaspoons brown sugar
1 dash fish sauce
½ medium jalapeno chile pepper, seeded and diced
1 cup basil leaves, chopped
½ cup slivered almonds

Polenta is coarsely ground yellow corn meal and is an essential ingredient of Northern Italian cuisine. Polenta is a great gluten-free substitute as a starchy side dish. We recommend sourcing organic polenta whenever possible since most of the non-organic corn comes from genetically modified crops. Cornmeal supplies a significant amount of fiber, and B vitamins as well as vitamin C and an antioxidant called xeazanthin, which may help protect against macular degeneration.

Serves 4

1 teaspoon salt
6 cups water
1 cup polenta
½ cup grated Parmesan, divided
1 generous pinch of cayenne pepper
vegetable oil cooking spray
2 cloves garlic, chopped
2 tablespoons chopped fresh oregano
2 tablespoons fresh lemon juice
1 tablespoon balsamic vinegar
1 tablespoon olive oil
1 zucchini, cut in half moon shapes
1 medium onion, peeled and quartered
1 small eggplant trimmed and halved
2 bell peppers, seeded and quartered
4 roma tomatoes rinsed and quartered
1 medium-large yellow squash (about pound), cut into half moons

Sauce
1 cup roasted red bell peppers drained (about 10 ounces)
2 tablespoons feta cheese
1 tablespoon balsamic vinegar
¼ teaspoon garlic powder
¼ teaspoon chopped rosemary

Per Serving:
450 Calories;
10g Fat (4g sat);
16g Protein;
77g Carbohydrate;
14g Dietary Fiber;
16mg Cholesterol;
790mg Sodium.

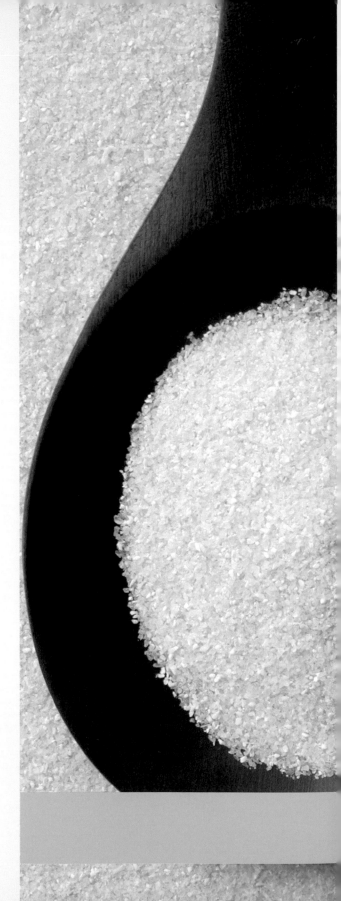

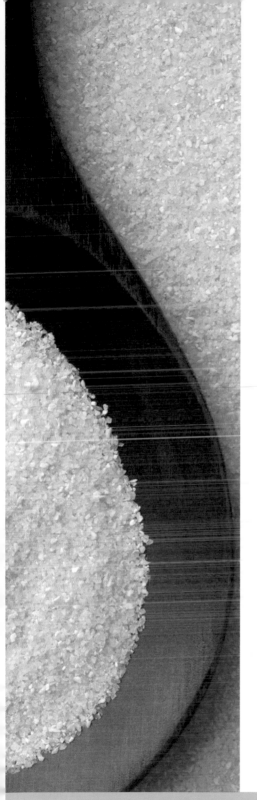

Bring 3 cups water and 1 teaspoon of salt to a boil in a medium-sized heavy saucepan. Have 3 additional cups of hot water simmering close by. Pour the polenta in a steady stream, whisking continuously to prevent the lumps from forming.

Reduce heat to medium-low and simmer, whisking frequently, until polenta starts to thicken. As it begins to get thicker, switch from a whisk to a wooden spoon. Stir in an additional cup of water and continue to stir. Press out any lumps with the back of the spoon. As the polenta thickens it will start to pull away from the sides of the pot. Taste the polenta from time to time to check for consistency (the timing will depend on the degree of coarseness of the polenta used). Our experience with polenta is that it takes around 30 minutes but it can vary as much as 15 minutes to an hour. Add more water if the polenta is pulling away from the sides but is still not tender and creamy. When it becomes creamy, stir in ¼ cup Parmesan cheese, a pinch of cayenne and about a ¼ teaspoon of sea salt. Keep stirring until it returns to creamy consistency.

Coat a 9-inch pie plate (or cast iron skillet) with cooking spray. Carefully pour polenta into pie plate, smooth it down and allow it to cool about 15 minutes.

Combine all ingredients for roasted red pepper sauce in a blender or food processor and blend until smooth. Place in a small pot, cover and heat over very low heat. Be careful that it doesn't boil. If it starts to simmer, remove from heat and keep covered.

Preheat broiler. Prepare a large baking sheet by lining it with aluminum foil or an even coating of cooking oil spray. Add chopped vegetables to a medium size bowl. In a separate smaller bowl, whisk together garlic, oregano, vinegar, lemon juice, oil, salt, and pepper. Pour on top of vegetables and toss well. Arrange vegetables on baking sheet in a single layer. Broil vegetables about 4 inches from heat until tender and slightly charred, 3 to 5 minutes on each side.

Sprinkle polenta with remaining ¼ cup Parmesan. Broil polenta in pie plate until golden brown, about 2 to 3 minutes. Remove from oven and allow to cool for just a few minutes. Then cut polenta into 8 triangles. Serve 2 polenta triangles with vegetables and top with roasted pepper sauce. Serve any remaining sauce on the side.

Inspired Polenta

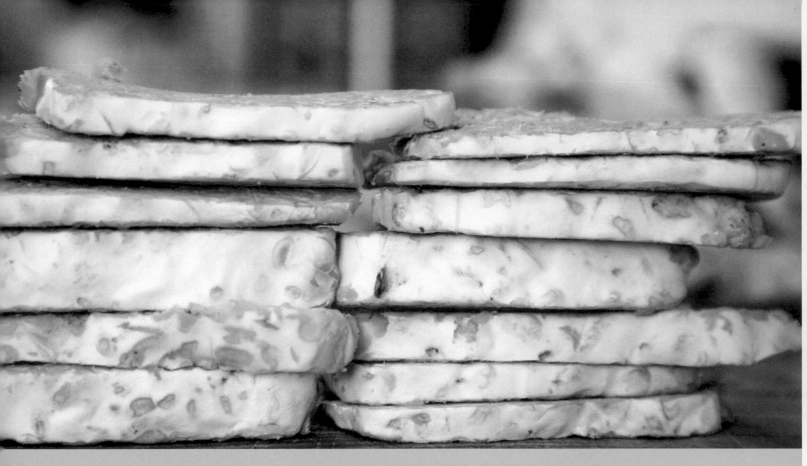

Simply Tempeh

Whisk together all ingredients except the tempeh and pickled ginger in a nonreactive dish. Add Tempeh and refrigerate for at least 2 hours and up to 2 days.

When you are ready to cook the tempeh, preheat the oven to 375°F. Put the marinated tempeh on a nonstick baking pan or glass dish coated with cooking spray. Bake for about 15 minutes on one side then turn the tempeh pieces over and bake for 10 to 12 minutes on the other side. Remove from oven and serve immediately garnished with pickled ginger or save for use on salads or sandwiches.

Alternatively you can cut the marinated tempeh into bite sized cubes and stir-fry them along with chopped vegetables, using a little of the leftover marinade to flavor the stir-fry. Serve over brown rice and sprinkle with sunflower seeds.

Serves 4

1 tablespoon fresh minced ginger
2 cloves garlic, minced or pressed
2 tablespoons tamari soy sauce
1 tablespoon vinegar
8 ounces tempeh, cut into 4 to 8
   slices, depending on how you
   want to use it
2 slices pickled ginger (optional)

Per Serving:
155 Calories;
5g Fat (1g sat);
12g Protein;
19g Carbohydrate;
1g Dietary Fiber;
0mg Cholesterol;
310mg Sodium.

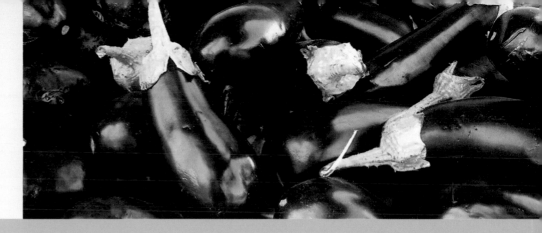

For the carb-conscious or gluten-intolerant this is a fun twist on lasagna – chock full of lycopene, vitamins and minerals.

Serves 8 to 10

Noodleless Veggie Lasagna

1 medium eggplant, sliced
   lengthwise
2 medium zucchini, sliced
   lengthwise
1 medium red bell pepper, seeded
   and chopped horizontally
2 medium yellow squash
1 cup butternut squash, peeled,
   seeded and thinly sliced (you
   can use a mandolin or vegetable
   peeler for this)
1 garlic clove, minced
1 cup sliced mushrooms
olive oil spray
25½ ounces tomato sauce or
   marinara
2 tablespoons 3 cheese blend **
15 ounces low fat ricotta **
15 ounces lowfat cottage cheese **
2 tablespoons fresh basil
½ cup lowfat mozzarella cheese,
   sliced **
sea salt and pepper to taste

Per Serving:
206 Calories;
6g Fat (3g sat)
21g Carbohydrate;
5g Dietary Fiber;
28mg Cholesterol;
673mg Sodium.

Rinse, seed (if necessary) and slice all vegetables (eggplant, zucchini, bell pepper, yellow squash, butternut squash). Set aside these vegetables (note: do not add to sauce). Lightly coat with olive oil spray and if desired sprinkle with a little sea salt. You can pre-grill or broil these veggies for a little extra flavor before adding to lasagna.

Heat a medium size skillet over medium high heat and coat with cooking spray. Add garlic and mushrooms and stir frequently until mushrooms start to brown and "sweat." Add tomato sauce, any additional vegetables (ends from zucchini and bell pepper or spinach) that you would like.

Preheat oven to 350°F.

In a medium size bowl, combine ricotta and cottage cheese.

In a large baking dish (approximately 13 x 9 inches), add about ¼ cup of the pasta sauce and spread around so it lightly coats the entire bottom of the dish. On top of this, layer the sliced eggplant and butternut squash. Spoon about half the ricotta and cottage cheese mixture on top of this layer. Follow with about ½ the remaining pasta sauce mixture on top of this layer. Next layer is the green and yellow squashes. Top again with ricotta and cottage cheese mixture and remaining pasta sauce. Top this off with slices of fresh mozzarella, fresh basil and sliced red bell pepper. Sprinkle with 2 tablespoons 3 cheese blend. Bake for 40 minutes.

After removing from oven, allow to sit for at least 10 minutes before cutting.

** for lower fat version you can reduce the amount of total cheese in this recipe.

191

This recipe for tofu is great because you can use it to make just about anything. You can serve this tofu along side rice and vegetables, use it on a sandwich or on top of salads. You can even add it to soups to boost the protein content.

Serves 4

Per Serving:
121 Calories;
9g Fat (1g sat);
10g Protein;
3g Carbohydrate;
1g Dietary Fiber;
0mg Cholesterol;
260mg Sodium.

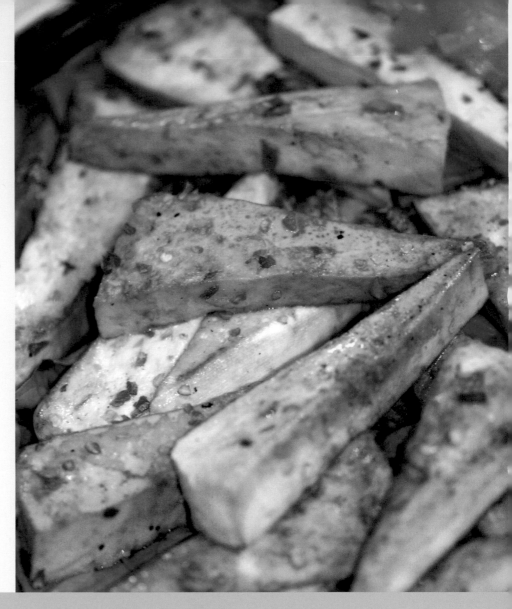

Simply Tofu

1 tablespoon sesame oil
½ teaspoon dried red pepper
1 teaspoon fresh ginger, minced
1 clove garlic, minced
1 tablespoon tamari soy sauce, divided
16 ounces firm tofu, cut into triangles**

Heat sesame oil in a fry pan (cast iron if available), add ½ teaspoon dried red pepper, fresh ginger, and garlic. Cook and stir over medium heat for 2 to 3 minutes. Add tofu to pan and drizzle tamari on top. Pan sear until lightly browned.

**To cut into triangles, first slice into rectangles then cut across diagonally into triangles.

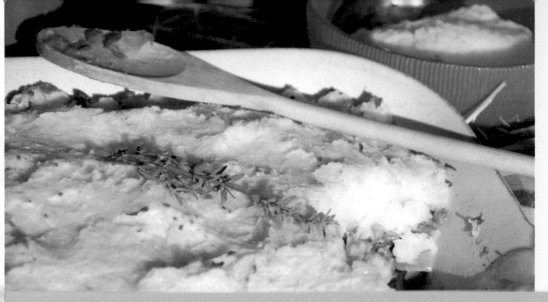

When we were baking for the Common Sense café, one of our favorite menu items was Shepherd's Pie. We ate Shepherd's Pie every night for months. A great choice for vegans and omnivores alike.

Serves 8

Big Horn Shepherd's Pie

Cook potatoes in boiling water for about 25 minutes until tender. Drain well and set aside.

Pick over lentils to remove any tiny rocks, debris or shriveled lentils. Rinse and drain the lentils and then add them to a medium pot, add 1 cup vegetable broth plus 1 cup of water. Bring to a boil for a few minutes then reduce heat and simmer until the lentils are tender - about 30 minutes. If the lentils are not fully soft add a bit more vegetable broth.

While the lentils are cooking, sauté onion, garlic, and carrots in olive oil until the onions are translucent and the carrots start to become tender, about 10 minutes. Remove from heat then stir in green peas, thyme, salt and pepper. When lentils are done cooking, stir them into this mixture.

Preheat oven to 350°F. Mash potatoes or use an electric beater to whip them up, adding milk, butter (or oil), cheese, salt, pepper, and cayenne. For additional spice you can add another dash of cayenne to the potato mixture.

Transfer lentil mixture to a medium size casserole dish (3 or 3.5 quart) that has been coated with cooking oil spray. Spoon mashed potato mixture on top of the lentils so that the potatoes are evenly distributed across the lentils. Bake for 30 minutes. Allow to sit for 5 minutes before serving.

6 medium red potatoes, about 1½ pounds
1 cup lentils
2 cups low sodium vegetable broth, divided
2 tablespoons olive oil
1 large chopped onions
2 cloves garlic cloves, minced
2 large carrots, roughly chopped
½ cup frozen peas
½ teaspoon thyme, or rosemary
¼ teaspoon sea salt
¼ teaspoon pepper
½ cup lowfat 2% milk
2 tablespoons butter or olive oil
½ cup grated Parmesan cheese
additional salt and pepper to taste
1 pinch of cayenne pepper

Per Serving:
245 Calories;
8g Fat (3g sat);
14g Protein;
30g Carbohydrate;
10g Dietary Fiber;
13mg Cholesterol;
341mg Sodium.

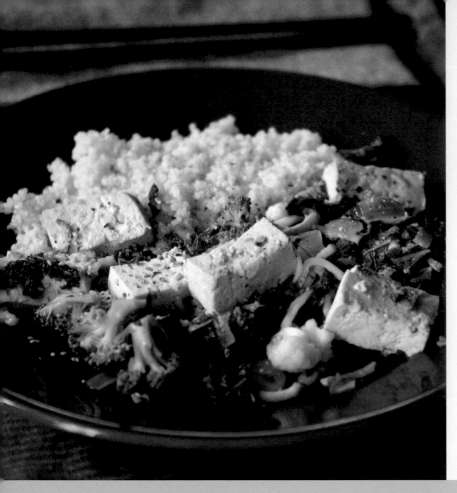

For seasoned vegetarians or tofu-phobics, this is an easy recipe to grasp and delicious in your meal rotation repertoire.

Serves 4

Per Serving:
268 Calories;
14g Fat (2g sat);
19g Protein;
22g Carbohydrate;
2g Dietary Fiber;
0mg Cholesterol;
272mg Sodium.

Tofu (or Tempeh) Stir-fry

Sauté tempeh, olive oil, garlic, ginger, and onion about 4 minutes over medium high heat in nonstick skillet or wok. Add remaining ingredients, except sesame seeds, and stir-fry about 10 minutes or until vegetables are cooked al dente. Serve with rice, quinoa, or whole grain pasta. Sprinkle with sesame seeds if desired.

*Note: If you are using tofu, first press out excess moisture by placing block of tofu on a plate with a clean dish towel or paper towels. Place an additional dish-towel or paper towel on top of the tofu and then a heavy book on top of that to press out the moisture.

12 ounces tempeh or firm tofu*, chopped or diced
2 tablespoons olive oil
1 clove garlic, chopped
1 teaspoon ginger, minced
½ cup onion, diced
1 cup asparagus spears, chopped
1 cup kale, rinsed and chopped
½ cup zucchini, chopped or grated
1 whole carrot, sliced
1 tablespoon tamari soy sauce
2 tablespoons water
other vegetables of choice
4 tablespoons sesame seeds (optional)

Our kids enjoy this recipe because it reminds them of eating out at an Asian restaurant. For them it is one of the "safest" things on the menu. We like it for the balanced protein, complex carbohydrates, and phytosterols, which may help reduce the risk of heart disease.

Serves 4

Per Serving:
286 Calories;
9g Fat (2g sat);
13g Protein;
38g Carbohydrate;
5g Dietary Fiber;
106mg Cholesterol;
617mg Sodium.

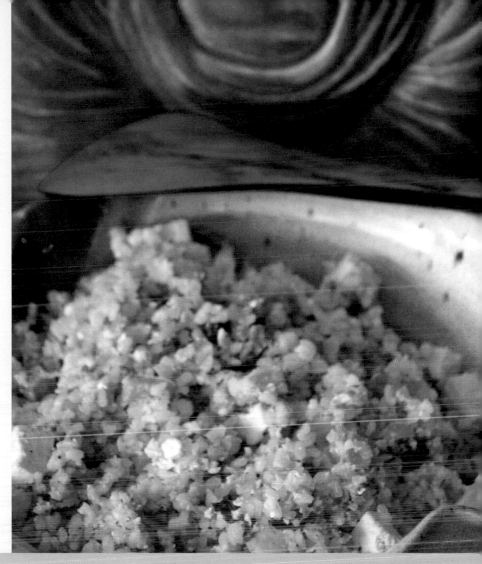

Four Corners Fried Rice

1 tablespoon olive oil
1 tablespoon fresh ginger, grated or minced
1 clove garlic, minced
1 cup firm tofu, drained (with excess water pressed out) and cubed
2 cups assorted vegetables (broccoli, cauliflower, asparagus, zucchini), fine dice
2 cups cooked brown rice
2 tablespoons teriyaki sauce (we use gluten-free teriyaki sauce by San-J)
2 eggs, slightly beaten

Heat the oil in a wok or large skillet over medium-high heat. Add the ginger and garlic and stir-fry about one minute. Add drained tofu and stir-fry another 3 minutes until the tofu and ginger and garlic are lightly browned. Add the mixed vegetables and continue to cook and stir-fry another 3 to 4 minutes. Stir in the cooked rice and teriyaki sauce.

Make a well in the center of the rice mixture and pour in the eggs. Cook the eggs until almost set before stirring them into the rice. Serve warm.

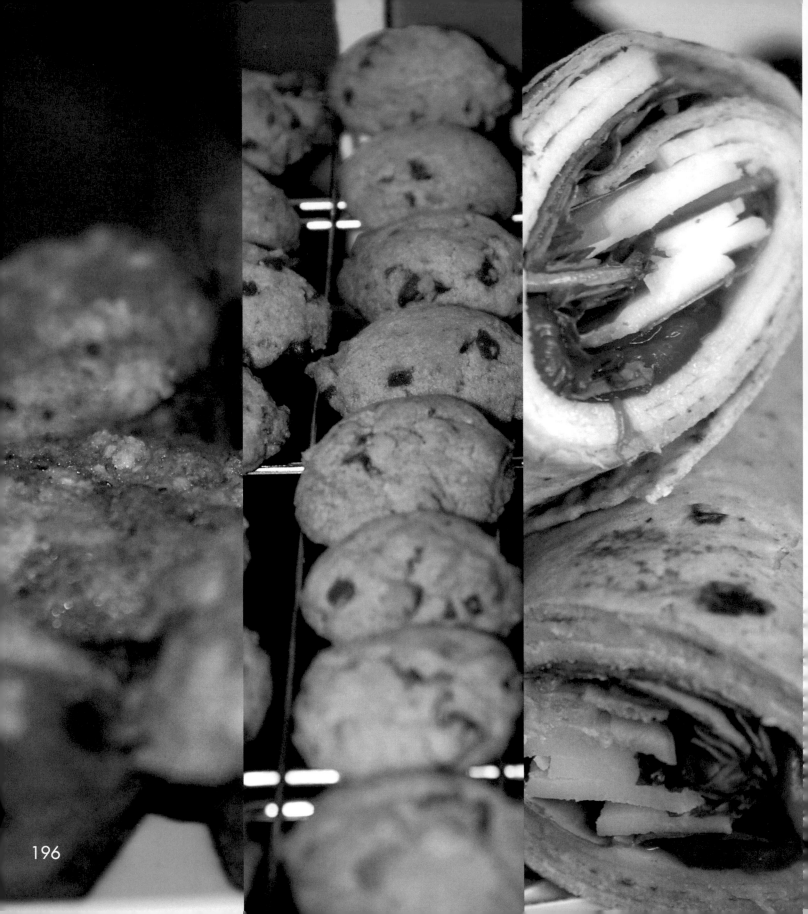

*To be yourself in a world that is constantly trying to make
you something else is the greatest accomplishment. ~ Ralph Waldo Emerson*

Fit Kids

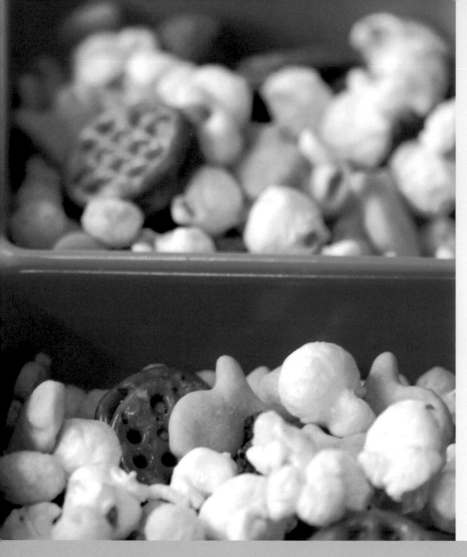

Though this mix varies about as often as she makes it, this is a snapshot of a fun kid's trail mix that will make your house the favorite place to hit up for snacks! She will usually use a combination of low-sugar cereal with whole grain pretzels, some kind of nut, a little sweetness from chocolate or dried fruit and occasionally some whole grain crackers. This particular batch is a little higher drama. You may want to consider going with either the raisins or the chocolate – or omitting the kettle corn and adding raw almonds instead. Give the kids a little freedom and teach them the importance of balance.

Serves about 12

Dakota's Happy Trails Mix

Combine all of the above ingredients in a large bowl. Stir or toss together gently with a large wooden mixing spoon. Serve in small bowls or use a measuring cup to measure one cup into snack-sized baggies to aid in portion control.

Per Serving:
338 Calories;
11g Fat (3g sat);
6g Protein;
54g Carbohydrate;
3g Dietary Fiber;
1mg Cholesterol;
287mg Sodium.

1 cup Panda Puffs cereal (Nature's Path) (or sub honey nut O's)
1 cup peanut butter pretzels (these are pretzels filled with peanut butter)
½ cup chocolate covered peanuts (or sub chocolate chips)
½ cup organic raisins
1 cup kettle corn
1 cup whole grain cheddar Goldfish® or Annie's Cheddar Bunnies

Choco Gramananas

Elli started whipping these little numbers up in preschool and by the time she hit second grade, she had mastered them. The surprising combination of the lemon zest and the chocolate syrup really works. We usually choose an organic chocolate syrup from either Ahlaska or Santa Cruz Organic. Unlike most conventional brands the organic brands contain no high fructose corn syrup.

Serves 2

1 medium banana
2 graham crackers
½ teaspoon lemon zest
1 tablespoon chocolate syrup
4 mint leaves
2 edible flowers

Slice banana into ½ inch rounds. Set aside.

Crush graham crackers in a sealed sandwich baggie until they are made into little crumbs.

Carefully add sliced banana into baggie with graham crackers and gently shake until the bananas are well coated with graham crumbs.

Divide bananas onto two small plates or bowls. Sprinkle with ¼ teaspoon of lemon zest and drizzle with chocolate sauce. Garnish with fresh mint and edible flowers.

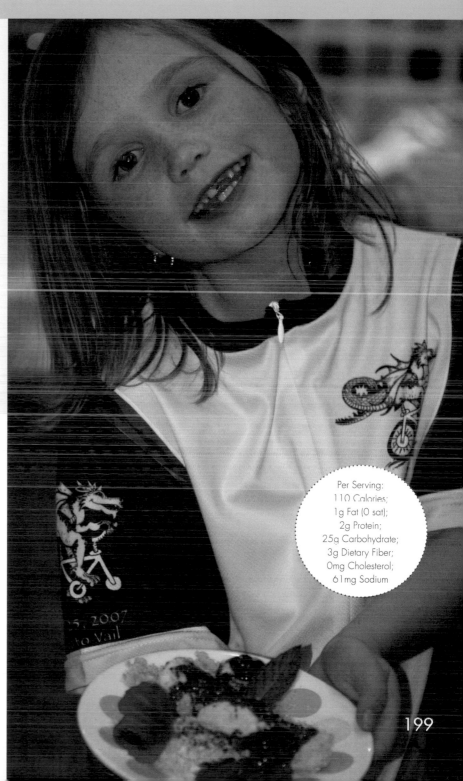

Per Serving:
110 Calories;
1g Fat (0 sat);
2g Protein;
25g Carbohydrate;
3g Dietary Fiber;
0mg Cholesterol;
61mg Sodium

Traditional grilled cheese sandwiches as we recall are made with white bread, American cheese and a lot of butter. Today's American cheese is generally no longer made from a blend of all-natural cheeses, but instead is manufactured from a combination of things including milk, whey, milk fat, milk protein concentrate, whey protein concentrate, and salt. It therefore does not meet the legal definition of cheese – not that there's anything wrong with that, but still we're offering a real "cheesy" version of the classic with more fiber and protein.

Serves 1

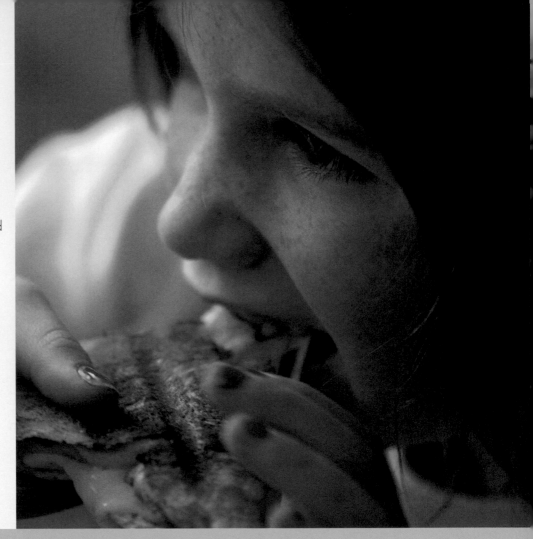

Grilled Cheese Makeover

2 slices whole wheat bread
1 slice organic Monterey Jack cheese
1 slice provolone cheese
cooking oil spray

Per Serving:
350 Calories;
11g Fat (6g sat);
20g Protein;
38g Carbohydrate;
6g Dietary Fiber;
30mg Cholesterol;
640mg Sodium.

Lightly coat one side of each piece of bread with cooking oil spray. Plug in an electric Panini sandwich press, or prepare a small nonstick skillet by placing it over medium heat. Layer the cheese between the two pieces of bread with the sides that have been coated with cooking oil spray facing out.

Grill on each side for about 2 to 3 minutes or for a total of 3 to 4 minutes on the Panini press. Be careful removing sandwich from the grill or pan and be sure to unplug or turn off the stove.

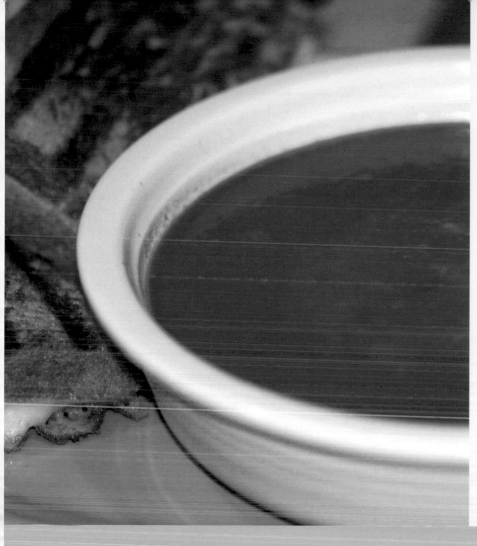

We put this recipe in our kids section because our kids love it — especially with a side of grilled cheese. Still we recommend adult supervision for kids under 12 due to the work on the stove and transferring of hot liquids to a blender or food processor. Kids love the stirring part so be sure to include them with that! This soup is loaded with lycopene — with absorption enhanced by the olive oil.

Serves 6

Per Serving.
218 Calories;
12g Fat (5g sat);
13g Protein;
18g Carbohydrate;
6g Dietary Fiber;
21mg Cholesterol;
453mg Sodium.

Creamy Tomato Soup

Sauté onion in olive oil and butter for 3 minutes or until transparent. Add garlic and tomatoes, continuing to sauté over medium heat for three to five minutes. Add broth. Cook, stirring constantly, for one minute. Stir in pepper, honey, and basil. Cook for another 5 minutes. Remove from heat and allow to cool slightly before blending. Transfer to a food processor or blender and purée until smooth.

Return puréed ingredients to soup pot and turn heat on low. When soup just starts to simmer, turn off heat and stir in cream. Serve hot or chilled.

1 tablespoon olive oil
1 tablespoon butter
1 medium onion, diced
1 garlic clove, chopped
8 medium ripe tomatoes, chopped
3 cups low sodium vegetable broth,
  or chicken broth
¼ teaspoon pepper
1 teaspoon honey, or brown sugar
1 teaspoon fresh basil, chopped plus
  more for garnish
¼ cup cream

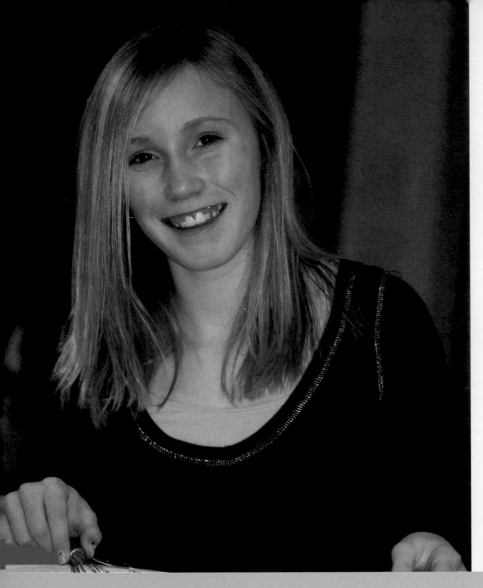

Our kids have always loved dipping vegetables into a Ranch-style dressing. Recently we healthified a favorite recipe and Dakota whipped it together for a fun gathering of friends. You can also use this on salads – whisk in a little extra buttermilk to thin it out and just toss it with your favorite greens.

About 10 servings

Dakota's Ranch Dip

Mix or whisk all ingredients together in a medium size bowl. Serve with tray of raw vegetables.

Per Serving:
49 Calories;
4g Fat (trace sat);
2g Protein;
2g Carbohydrate;
trace Dietary Fiber;
5mg Cholesterol;
106mg Sodium

1 cup lowfat mayonnaise
1 cup Greek-style nonfat yogurt
1 teaspoon garlic powder
1 teaspoon onion flakes
2 tablespoons lemon juice
2 tablespoons fresh parsley, finely chopped
2 tablespoons green onion, diced
¼ teaspoon sea salt
¼ teaspoon black pepper

For many years we have surrendered to the "beige diet" our daughter Elli has perfected. She loves most beige food – quesadillas, toast, cereal, and pasta. Elli's idea of the perfect meal is pasta - plain. We've found a way to add just enough flavor to it by combining some heart healthy olive oil with some decadent butter and fresh basil. Ideally add some protein to the pasta like a piece of string cheese, a few ounces of sliced chicken, or some crumbled tofu.

Serves 4

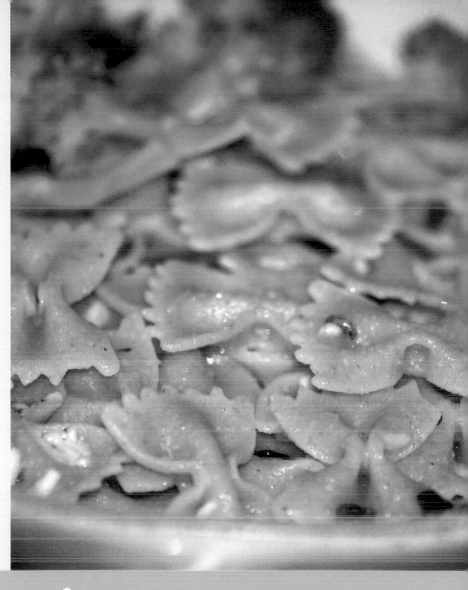

Elli's Perfect Pasta

8 ounces whole wheat bow tie pasta
1 tablespoon olive oil
1 tablespoon butter
½ teaspoon fresh basil
1 dash sea salt
1 dash pepper
4 tablespoons Parmesan cheese

2 cups cooked broccoli

Prepare pasta according to package directions. Drain and return back to the pot. Stir in butter and olive oil. Then stir in basil, salt and pepper.

Divide pasta into 4 serving bowls and sprinkle with 1 tablespoon of Parmesan cheese. Serve with a side of steamed broccoli.

Per Serving:
309 Calories,
9g Fat (3g sat);
13g Protein;
45g Carbohydrate;
8g Dietary Fiber;
12mg Cholesterol;
201mg Sodium.

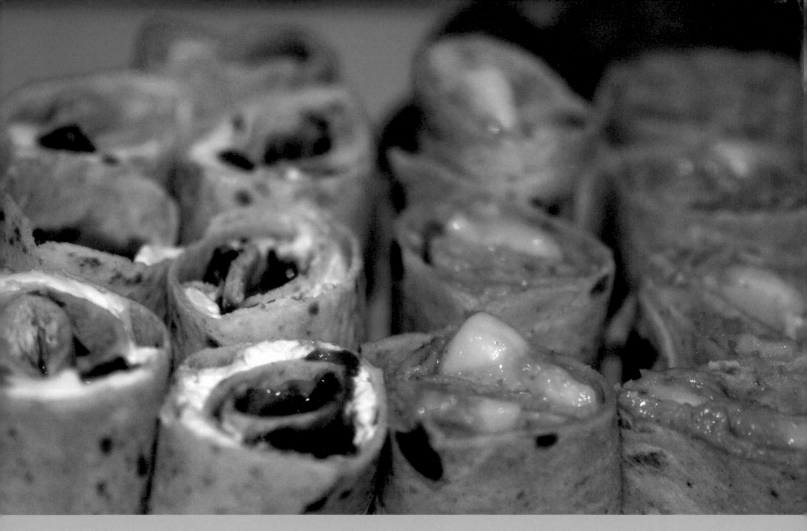

"Sushi-style" Roll Ups

Serves 2

Cream-cheese and Jelly version
2 whole wheat tortillas
3 tablespoons cream cheese
2 tablespoon raspberry jelly

Peanut Butter, Honey, and Banana version
2 whole wheat tortillas
2 tablespoons peanut butter
1 tablespoon honey
1 medium banana

204

Cream-cheese and Jelly version
Spread 1 ½ tablespoons cream cheese plus ½ tablespoon jelly across each tortilla. Roll up from one end and slice into ½ inch "rolls."

Peanut Butter, Honey, and Banana version
Spread 1 tablespoon peanut butter, ½ tablespoon honey and ½ banana slices on each tortilla. Roll up from one end and slice into ½ inch "rolls."

Per Serving:
216 Calories; 5g Fat (2g sat); 5g Protein; 39g Carbohydrate; 2g Dietary Fiber; 8mg Cholesterol; 430mg Sodium.

Per Serving:
322 Calories; 11g Fat (2g sat); 9g Protein; 52g Carbohydrate; 4g Dietary Fiber; 0mg Cholesterol; 456mg Sodium.

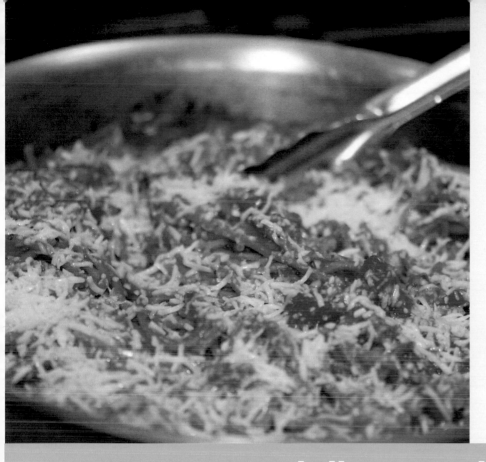

This is a really quick and easy main course. We often will add cut vegetables to the marinara sauce before adding the pasta. Vegetarians can substitute tofu or tempeh for the ground turkey, or leave it out altogether. We always recommend balancing out the carbohydrate load with some quality protein.

Serves 6

Skillet Spaghetti

Prepare spaghetti according to package directions. Drain. While the spaghetti is cooking, heat 1 tablespoon of olive oil over medium heat in a large cast-iron or other oven-safe skillet. Add turkey and brown it until cooked through, breaking apart any large clumps of ground turkey. Add marinara to the skillet with the cooked turkey. Reduce heat to low and stir so that the turkey is well mixed into the marinara.

Stir in drained spaghetti and mix well until all of the sauce is well incorporated into the spaghetti. Now, there are 2 ways of serving this. You can either stop here, divide the mixture onto serving plates, and top with 2 tablespoons of freshly grated Parmesan cheese – or – you can sprinkle all of the cheese on top of the spaghetti mixture and bake in a 350°F oven for 20 minutes, which will produce more of a crispy topping.

1 pound whole wheat (or gluten free)
* spaghetti, uncooked*
1 tablespoon olive oil
1 pound ground turkey breast
3 cups low sodium marinara
¾ cup Parmesan cheese, grated

Per Serving:
470 Calories;
10g Fat (2g sat);
29g Protein;
63g Carbohydrate;
3g Dietary Fiber;
47mg Cholesterol;
227mg Sodium.

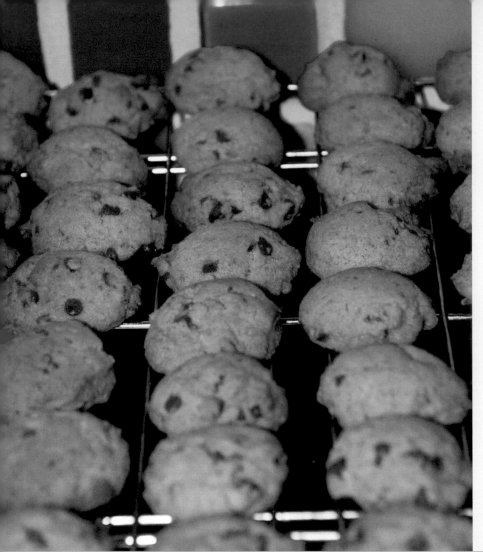

Our kids don't want anything other than chocolate chips in their cookies – no nuts, no raisins – you get the picture. We've cut a lot of the excess sugar and partially hydrogenated fat out of the traditional recipe by using an organic shortening (we use Spectrum) that is trans fat free. By using whole grain flour we also add a little bit of fiber to the cookies – a win/win all the way around. For a gluten-free version, substitute brown rice flour for the whole wheat pastry flour – it subs out quite nicely.

Makes 58 cookies

Per Serving
(2 cookies):
127 Calories; 7g Fat
(4g sat); 1g Protein;
16g Carbohydrate;
1g Dietary Fiber;
16mg Cholesterol;
101mg Sodium.

Mini Chippers

Preheat oven to 350°F.

In large bowl of an electric mixer, cream together butter, shortening and sugars. Beat in egg and vanilla. Combine flour, baking soda and salt; stir or beat into butter mixture, until well mixed. Stir in chocolate chips.

Drop by rounded teaspoonfuls, 2" apart, onto cookie sheets lined with parchment paper. Bake for about 9 to 10 minutes, just until edges are golden (centers will still be soft). Remove to wire racks to cool.

½ cup butter, softened
¼ cup organic shortening
½ cup packed brown sugar
½ cup maple sugar
1 egg
1 teaspoon vanilla
2 ¼ cups whole wheat pastry flour
1 teaspoon baking soda
¼ teaspoon salt
¾ cup miniature chocolate chips

Raspberry Orange Mighty Mini Muffins

When it comes time to bring snack to school for the entire class, or snacks for the soccer team, these are an easy choice. They also freeze well so you can pull out a few at a time and they make for a great mid-day snack with a cup of tea.

Makes 36 miniature muffins or 1 dozen regular size

For streusel topping:
3 tablespoons almonds
2 tablespoons flour
2 tablespoons brown sugar
1 teaspoon freshly grated orange zest
¼ teaspoon salt
2 tablespoons melted butter

For the muffins:
1 cup whole-wheat pastry flour
½ cup all-purpose flour
¼ cup ground flax seed
2 teaspoons baking powder
1 teaspoon baking soda
½ teaspoon cinnamon
¼ teaspoon salt
¼ cup brown sugar
1 teaspoon freshly grated orange zest
¼ cup canola oil
½ cup lowfat buttermilk
¼ cup fresh squeezed orange juice
1 large egg
1 teaspoon vanilla extract
½ cup raspberry fruit spread

Preheat oven to 375°F. Prepare muffin tins with either small paper or parchment liners (or silicone cup molds).

Grind almonds in a food processor or coffee grinder. Combine ground almonds with 2 tablespoons flour, 2 tablespoons brown sugar, 1 teaspoon orange zest and ¼ teaspoon salt. Stir in 2 tablespoons melted butter and continue to combine until mixture is well mixed. Set aside until ready to use.

In a large bowl, whisk whole-wheat pastry flour, ½ cup all-purpose flour, ground flax, baking powder, baking soda, cinnamon, and ¼ teaspoon salt.

In a medium size bowl, whisk together ¼ cup brown sugar, 1 teaspoon orange zest and ¼ cup oil with buttermilk, orange juice, egg and vanilla extract until well combined. Make a well in the center of the dry ingredients and pour in the wet ingredients; stir until just combined. Stir in raspberry fruit spread.

Divide the batter among the prepared muffin cups, being careful not to overfill. Sprinkle lightly with the streusel topping, and gently press into the batter.

Bake the muffins until golden brown and a wooden skewer inserted in the center comes out clean, about 15 minutes. Let cool in the pan for 10 minutes, and then transfer to a wire rack to cool for at least 10 minutes more before serving. The muffins are very moist and will be easier to remove from their muffin liners if they are completely cooled.

Per Serving:
66 Calories;
3g Fat (1g sat);
1g Protein;
8g Carbohydrate;
1g Dietary Fiber;
8mg Cholesterol;
105mg Sodium.

When our daughter Dakota decided to become a vegetarian we were of course very supportive. At the same time we encouraged her to get a little more creative with her diet and make sure to get adequate protein through vegetarian sources. This is one of those perfect meals that packs a great protein punch and is still fun, reminiscent of the original ground beef version. In all honesty, we prefer this version, hands down.

Serves 6

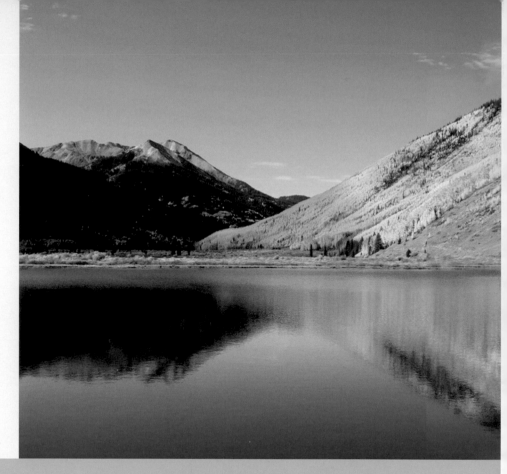

Tempeh Sloppy Joes

1 tablespoon olive oil
3 cups tempeh, chopped
¼ cup chopped onions
1 cup water
1 package organic sloppy Joe Seasoning
6 ounces tomato paste
2 tablespoons relish

Per Serving:
218 Calories;
9g Fat (1g sat);
17g Protein;
22g Carbohydrate;
1g Dietary Fiber;
0mg Cholesterol;
282mg Sodium

In a large skillet over medium heat, cook tempeh with onions in 1 tablespoon of olive oil. Use a spatula to break up the tempeh so that it is nice and crumbly. Reduce heat to low.

Combine Sloppy Joe mix with 1 cup of warm water. Whisk together until completely dissolved. Whisk in the tomato paste and then add this entire mixture to the tempeh and onions. Stir in relish.

Increase heat to medium and continue to stir until mixture begins to simmer. Once it starts to simmer, reduce heat and simmer for another 5 minutes. Serve on whole grain buns or English muffins.

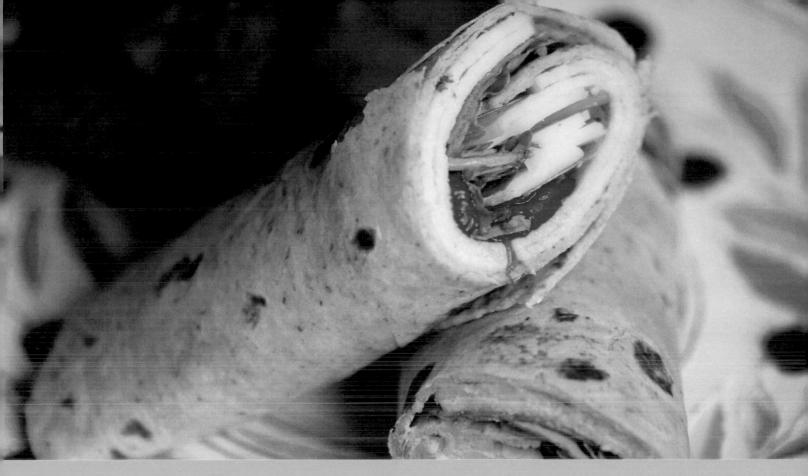

Whole Wheat Turkey Spinach Wrap

Lightly brush the majority of the inside of the wrap with pesto sauce using the back of a spoon. You can use a little bit of mayonnaise and/or mustard instead.

Place 2 ounces of sliced turkey into the center of each wrap. Add ¼ of the spinach leaves into the center of each tortilla. Top with a layer of red bell pepper strips. Sprinkle with a tablespoon of shredded cheese. Gently roll or fold tortilla into a burrito-like roll, starting at one end and rolling to the other. Cut in half for easier handling.

Serves 4

4 Low Carb Whole Wheat Wraps (or tortillas)
8 ounces nitrate-free roasted turkey
 breast (We like Applegate Farms)
2 teaspoons pesto sauce (p. 246)
½ cup roasted red pepper, cut into thin strips
4 ounces spinach leaves
4 organic provolone slices

Per Serving:
171 Calories;
10g Fat (4g sat);
14g Protein;
20g Carbohydrate;
13g Dietary Fiber;
16mg Cholesterol;
475mg Sodium.

209

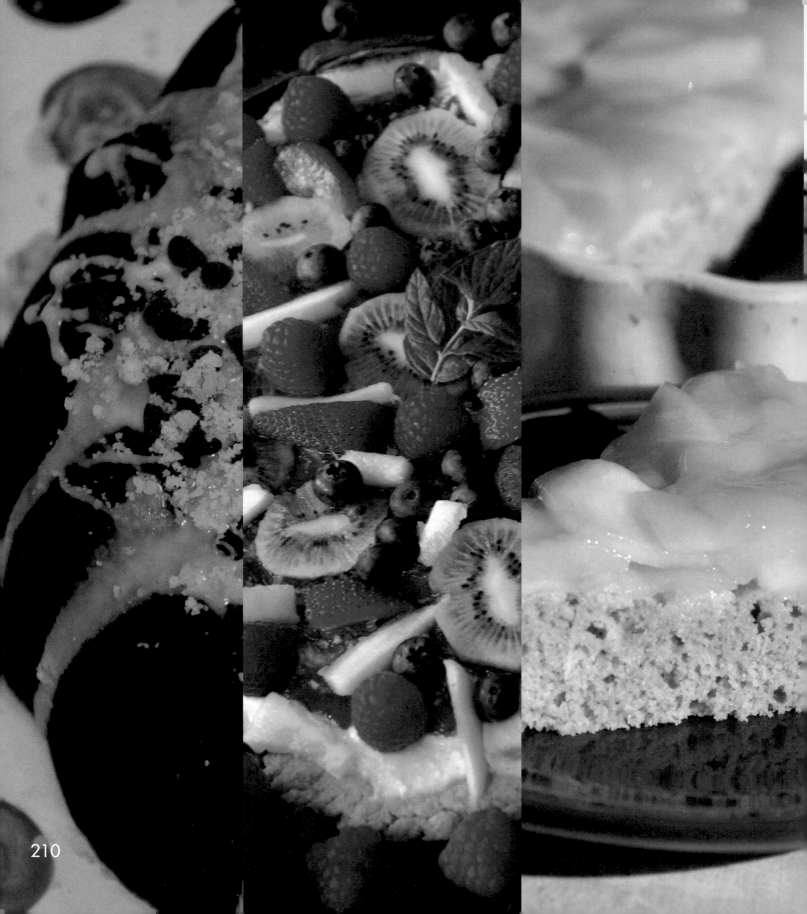

Forget love, I'd rather fall in chocolate. ~ Author Unknown

Decadence

Time for true confessions. For as much as we are health fanatics, we must admit that we love a great dessert. I've always been a baker (Deb talking). My love affair with baked goods began sometime in high school. Although I confess to eating more Hostess Apple Pies for lunch than I care to admit, I will say that I learned the fine art of healthy substitutions during my late teen years. Learning how to replace all the butter, sugar, and white flour in a recipe takes a bit of time, but once you get it, there's no end to the fun you can have with a basic recipe – you'll see that in our chocolate chip oatmeal cookies. Once I hit college, I further experimented with adding things like oat bran and flax seed to my baked goods. Of course once we partnered with the Common Sense café, baking became as much a nightly ritual as it was a nightly necessity.

Conscious Crumble

When we would go back to Maine to visit James' dad in the summer, one of the things we loved to do was hop on "Papa's scooter" and head down to the little store where they sold "Bumbleberry" pies. These were something from heaven and contained everything under the sun, including apples and berries, and a brown sugar oaty topping. This apple crumble is equally as delicious and versatile – in that just add a few blueberries, raspberries, blackberries, or strawberries and you've got yourself a bumbleberry pie.

Serves 6

Crust:
1 cup organic whole wheat pastry or brown rice flour
3 tablespoons ghee, canola oil or butter
3 tablespoons ice water

Filling:
6 cups Granny Smith apples peeled, cored, and chopped
1 tablespoon cinnamon
¼ teaspoon nutmeg
2 tablespoons lemon juice
2 tablespoons organic sugar or maple sugar

Nut crumb topping:
3 tablespoons butter
⅓ cup brown sugar or maple sugar
1 cup finely chopped walnuts
¼ cup flour
½ cup oats

Preheat oven to 325°F. To prepare crust, combine flour, ghee and water with a pastry cutter or food processor until mixture forms a ball. Roll out with rolling pin and place in greased pie shell.

Prepare apples and combine with other filling ingredients and set aside.

For topping, melt butter in small pan. Add brown sugar, walnuts, oats and flour and mix until crumbs form.

Spoon the apple filling into the piecrust and sprinkle with the crumb topping. Place pie pan on a cookie sheet and bake at 325°F for about an hour.

Per Serving:
372 Calories;
19g Fat (7g sat);
8g Protein;
47g Carbohydrate;
6g Dietary Fiber;
25mg Cholesterol;
49mg Sodium.

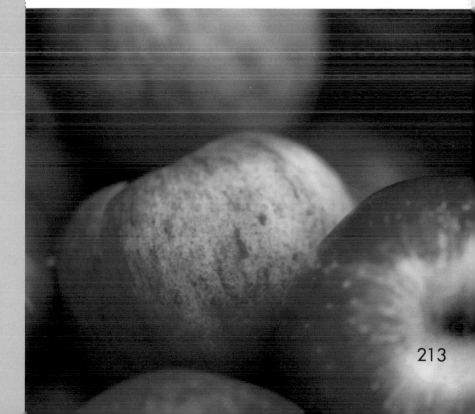

213

If you're wondering what to do with an abundance of fall fruit, this is a terrific cake. You can use all apples or all pears or both and either way you'll still have a fantastic cake. Both pears and apples are great sources of vitamin C and dietary fiber.

Serves 10

215 Calories;
5g Fat (2g sat);
4g Protein;
39g Carbohydrate;
3g Dietary Fiber;
71mg Cholesterol;
185mg Sodium.

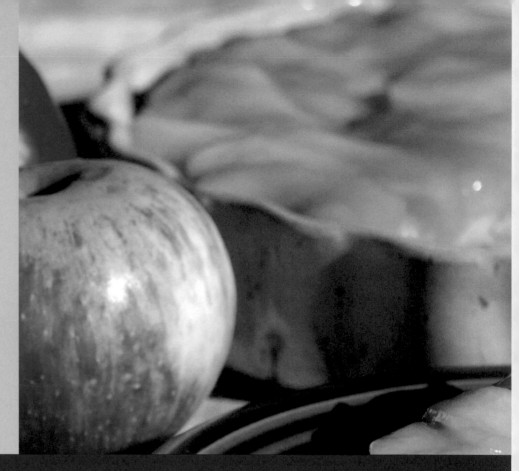

Apple-Pear Cake (Gluten-free)

1½ cups brown rice flour
2 teaspoons baking powder
½ teaspoon baking soda
½ teaspoon cinnamon
3 egg yolks
2 tablespoons ghee, melted
¼ cup maple syrup
2 teaspoons vanilla flavoring or extract
(if you need to avoid gluten, be sure to check the label)
3 egg whites
2 pears, cored, peeled and sliced
2 apples, cored, peeled and sliced
1 cup pear juice, or apple juice
2 tablespoons maple syrup

Preheat oven to 350°F. Lightly coat an 8-inch square or round baking dish with cooking oil spray. Mix together dry ingredients. In a separate bowl beat egg yolks, melted ghee, maple syrup and vanilla extract. Add this mixture to the flour mixture. In another bowl, beat egg whites until stiff. Fold into cake batter. Add cake batter to pan and bake for 20 minutes. Allow to cool on wire rack.

Combine sliced apples and pears with pear juice and maple syrup in a skillet and simmer until the liquid becomes thicker and the fruit is soft but not mushy.

Arrange cooked fruit over cake and then spoon some of the remaining liquid on top as a glaze.

214

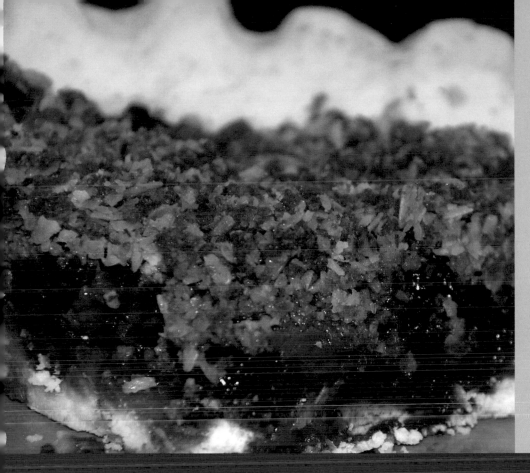

Dinner at the Rouse-House isn't complete without a homemade Berry Crisp. It was almost difficult to put this one on paper since we always just put it together with whatever berries we have on hand. Sometimes we'll make it with a crust and sometimes without. Occasionally we'll put the crust on top and call it a crumble! Either way, we usually always top it with yogurt or when feeling more indulgent, homemade whipped cream! If you make it without the prepared pie crust then the fat content will be considerably lower. It's like a quiche compared to a fritatta.

Serves 8

Berry Crisp

Preheat oven to 350°F. Combine berries in a large mixing bowl. Sprinkle with sugar and toss lightly. In a small bowl, stir together lemon juice and cornstarch. Pour this mixture over the berries and toss gently to coat.

Pour or spoon berries into prepared pie crust. (Remember, you can make this crisp crust-free)

Combine walnuts, flour, oats, brown sugar and butter in the bowl of food processor fitted with S-shaped cutting blade.
Pulse ingredients together until well combined.
Sprinkle crumb mixture evenly over berries.

Bake for about 35 to 40 minutes. Allow to cool at least 15 minutes before slicing.

Per Serving:
308 Calories;
16g Fat (6g sat);
5g Protein;
38g Carbohydrate;
4g Dietary Fiber;
16mg Cholesterol;
166mg Sodium.

2 tablespoons sugar
2 tablespoons fresh lemon juice
1 tablespoon cornstarch
2 cups fresh blueberries
2 cups fresh strawberries, sliced
1 cup fresh raspberries
1 prepared pie crust, whole wheat
   or gluten-free
½ cup chopped walnuts, or pecans
½ cup brown rice flour
½ cup oats, rolled (raw)
¼ cup brown sugar
4 tablespoons melted butter

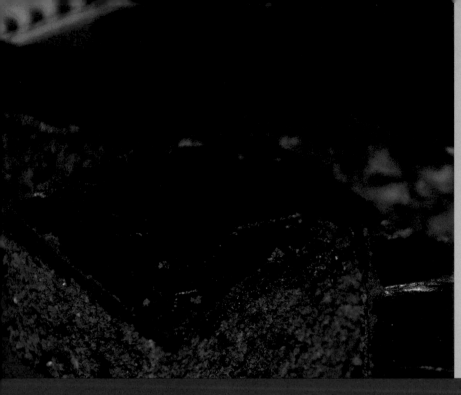

We've had great feedback on these decadent brownies. They are just sweet and rich enough to know that you are having something indulgent, yet they are also fortified with heart healthy flax, walnuts, and of course the cocoa power, which is also rich in antioxidants. The frosting is optional, so if you want a less "dramatic" version you can omit the frosting and top with a dollop of fresh whipped cream and berries.

Makes about 20 brownies

Mud Season Brownies

Preheat oven to 350°F. Mix together dry ingredients (excluding nuts). Melt ¼ cup butter and whisk it together with applesauce, eggs and vanilla. Add wet ingredients to dry and mix all ingredients together by hand adding chopped walnuts towards the end.

Pour into greased 8 × 11-inch baking pan, clear glass works best. Bake for 30 minutes.

If you want to frost the brownies for added decadence, combine chocolate chips with butter in a small saucepan over low heat (or use a double-boiler). Add milk (may need to use a little more than 2 tablespoons) and mix to smooth consistency. Whisk in powdered sugar until completely mixed in and then spread frosting on top of cooled brownies.

Per Brownie:
227 Calories;
12g Fat (6g sat);
4g Protein;
30g Carbohydrate;
2g Dietary Fiber;
58mg Cholesterol;
174mg Sodium.

Brownies:
1 cup whole wheat pastry flour
½ cup all purpose flour
2 tablespoons flax seed, ground
¾ cup sugar or sucanat (naturally unprocessed sugar)
¾ teaspoon salt
¾ teaspoon baking powder
5 tablespoons cocoa powder
¼ cup butter (melted) (you can use canola oil or non-hydrogenated baking sticks if you prefer)
¼ cup applesauce
4 eggs
1½ teaspoons vanilla
½ cup walnuts, chopped (optional)

Frosting (optional):
1 cup semisweet chocolate chips
2 tablespoons butter
2 tablespoons lowfat 2% milk
1 cup powdered sugar

When we served this at James' 40th birthday party, it was a bigger hit than the festive chocolate cake. We often make it gluten free using coconut flour, rice flour, and tapioca flour – just be patient with the crust. Blueberries are high in antioxidant phytonutrients called anthocyanidins, which protect the eyes, enhance the effects of vitamin C, and prevent free-radical damage. A fun and summery dessert you can feel good about eating.

Serves 8

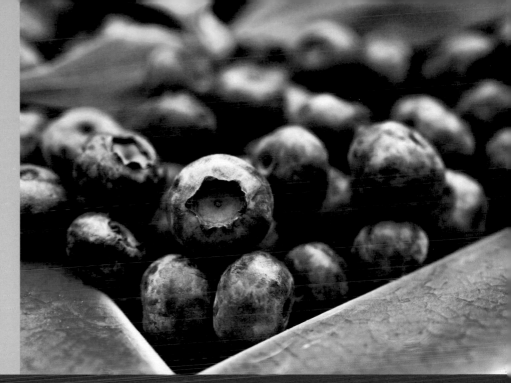

Blueberry Galette – a free form pie

1 cup all purpose flour
1 cup whole wheat pastry flour
¼ teaspoon sea salt
6 tablespoons butter
2 tablespoons lowfat 2% milk
2 tablespoons ice water

4 cups fresh blueberries
juice from ½ lemon
1 teaspoon cinnamon
1 teaspoon lemon peel
2 tablespoons honey
1 teaspoon arrowroot powder

Per Serving:
372 Calories;
18g Fat (11g sat);
8g Protein;
46g Carbohydrate;
5g Dietary Fiber;
47mg Cholesterol;
299mg Sodium

Preheat oven to 350°F. Combine flours and sea salt in food processor and pulse on high. Add butter and pulse until crumbly. Add milk and then ice water and blend on high until mixture forms a ball. Remove from food processor and refrigerate for 5 minutes.

Add blueberries to medium size bowl. Drizzle with lemon juice and stir. Add cinnamon and lemon peel, stir again. Add honey and arrowroot and stir until mixture is coated.

Place a large sheet of parchment paper on flat surface. Roll out pie dough on top of parchment into a large circle, 10 to 12 inches in diameter. Carefully slide dough and parchment onto large, flat baking sheet. Use a slotted spoon to add blueberry mixture to center of dough, leaving about 2 inches of plain dough surrounding the fruit. Then fold the sides of the pastry over the fruit and make sure to pinch down the sides so that the pastry stays in place. Bake for 40 to 45 minutes.

Remove from oven and let cool for at least 20 minutes before you remove it from the baking sheet.

217

This is the standard birthday and all-occasion cake for James. We've trimmed the fat, upped the fiber, made it gluten-free and absolutely fabulous. We often serve it frosting-free but for extra decadence a little cream cheese frosting is pretty awesome.

Serves 12

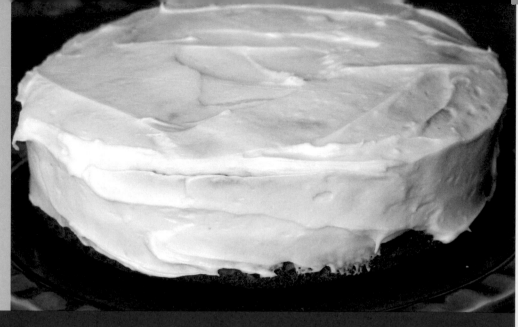

Ode to James Carrot Cake (Gluten-Free)

3 cups grated carrots
1 cup chopped walnuts
¼ cup ground flax seed
½ cup rolled oats
¾ cup canola oil
½ cup applesauce
1¼ cups sugar
6 large eggs
1½ teaspoons vanilla extract
1½ cups brown rice flour
½ cup coconut flour
¼ cup tapioca flour
1½ teaspoons baking soda
½ teaspoon salt
2 teaspoons cinnamon
½ teaspoon nutmeg
1 teaspoon ground ginger

Cream Cheese Frosting
4 ounces lowfat cream cheese
¼ cup butter
1 tablespoon grated lemon rind
1 teaspoon vanilla extract
3 ½ cups powdered sugar

Preheat oven to 375°F. Coat a 10-cup bundt or flute pan with cooking oil spray - or prepare two 9-inch cake rounds.

Toss together carrots through rolled oats.

Whisk together oil, applesauce, sugar, eggs, and vanilla extract.

In another bowl, whisk together flours, baking soda, salt, and spices.

Combine the dry ingredients with the oil-egg mixture. Stir in the carrot-nut mixture. Pour the batter into the prepared pan(s) and bake until golden brown and fully cooked through the center (about 30 to 35 minutes for cake rounds and 40 to 45 minutes for bundt). Cool the cake in the pan(s) on a wire rack until completely cool. Carefully remove from the baking pan and finish cooling completely on the wire rack. Allow to cool completely before frosting.

Cream Cheese Frosting
Beat together all ingredients with an electric mixer until smooth and creamy.

Per Serving: 427
Calories; 24g Fat
(2g sat); 9g Protein;
47g Carbohydrate; 4g Dietary Fiber;
106mg Cholesterol; 295mg Sodium.

Frosting
Per Serving: 97 Calories; 3g Fat
(2g sat); 1g Protein; 18g Carbohydrate;
trace Dietary Fiber;
8mg Cholesterol;
53mg Sodium.

218

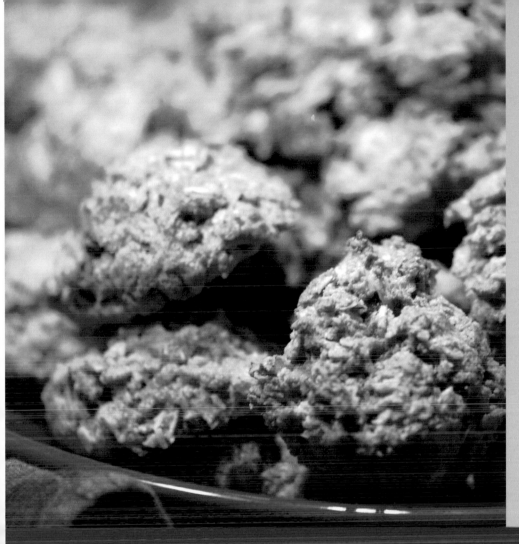

These are really fun cookies to make – you can shape them as big or small as you would like. They are slightly cakey from the oats and applesauce. Still a more heart-healthy version than the standard chocolate chip or oatmeal cookie – packed with flavor, antioxidants, and fiber.

Makes about 3 dozes

Per Serving:
298 Calories,
13g Fat (7g sat);
6g Protein;
43g Carbohydrate;
4g Dietary Fiber;
37mg Cholesterol;
177mg Sodium

Mindful Morsels

Preheat oven to 350°F. In a large mixing bowl, beat butter and sugar until light and fluffy. Add eggs, applesauce and vanilla and beat until smooth.

In a separate bowl, combine flour, baking soda, salt, and cinnamon. Add to butter and brown sugar mixture and beat until smooth and creamy.
Stir in oats, coconut and chocolate chips. Drop by rounded teaspoons onto nonstick cookie sheet lightly sprayed with cooking oil. Bake 10 minutes or until light brown.

Remove cookie sheet from oven and allow cookies to cool about 3 minutes before placing them on a wire rack to cool.

½ cup butter
¾ cup packed brown sugar
2 eggs
½ cup applesauce
2 teaspoons vanilla
1½ cups whole wheat pastry flour
1 teaspoon baking soda
¼ teaspoon salt
½ teaspoon cinnamon
3 cups oats
½ cup flaked coconut
½ cup chocolate chips

219

Celestial Bundt Cake

Preheat oven to 350°F and prepare a large Bundt cake pan by coating it evenly with cooking spray. Alternatively you can make a (9 x 13) sheet cake.

Whisk together flours, sugar, cocoa, baking powder and soda, spices and salt in a medium size bowl. In another bowl or in a stand up mixer, beat together buttermilk, pumpkin purée and brown sugar. Beat in eggs. Stir in oil, brown rice syrup, and vanilla. Gradually stir in the dry ingredients until just combined. Transfer the cake batter to the prepared pan.

Bake for an hour (convection ovens) to an hour and fifteen minutes. Cool completely on a wire rack. It is especially difficult to try and remove a bundt cake if it has not cooled completely. Once you have the cake removed, continue to cool on a wire rack before glazing. When ready to glaze, transfer cake to serving platter.

For the glaze: Combine the powdered sugar with 1 tablespoon of milk and whisk together until smooth. Drizzle the glaze over the top of the cake. Top with optional mini chocolate chips and/or chopped walnuts.

Per Serving (with added nuts and choc. chips): 218 Calories; 6g Fat (1g sat); 4g Protein; 41g Carbohydrate; 3g Dietary Fiber; 14mg Cholesterol; 228mg Sodium.

Per Serving (without added nuts and choc. chips): 205 Calories; 5g Fat (1g sat); 4g Protein; 40g Carbohydrate; 3g Dietary Fiber; 14mg Cholesterol; 227mg Sodium.

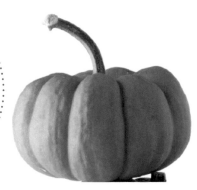

We first discovered this recipe in Eating Well magazine, one of our favorites. James featured it on 9news and it received rave reviews. We've cut the sugar a bit and made a few substitutions, but it is still full of flavor, flavonoids and heart healthy goodness. We like to serve it with homemade whipped cream.

Serves 16

Cake:
1 cup whole wheat flour
¾ cup whole wheat pastry flour
¾ cup sucanat (natural sugar)
¾ cup unsweetened cocoa powder
1½ teaspoons baking powder
1½ teaspoons baking soda
1 teaspoon cinnamon
¼ teaspoon ginger
¼ teaspoon nutmeg
¼ teaspoon salt
1 cup lowfat buttermilk
1 can (15 ounces) pumpkin purée
½ cup brown sugar
2 large eggs
¼ cup canola oil
¼ cup brown rice syrup or agave nectar or honey
1 tablespoon vanilla extract

Glaze:
½ cup powdered sugar
1 tablespoon lowfat milk
2 tablespoons walnuts - optional
2 tablespoons mini-chocolate chips - optional

220

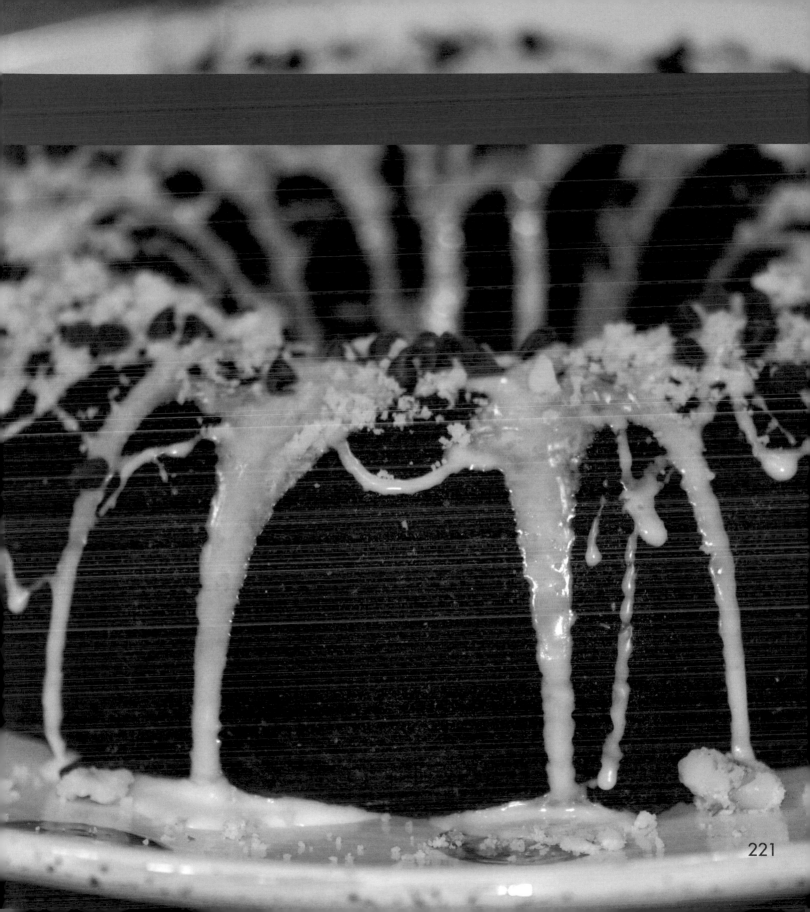

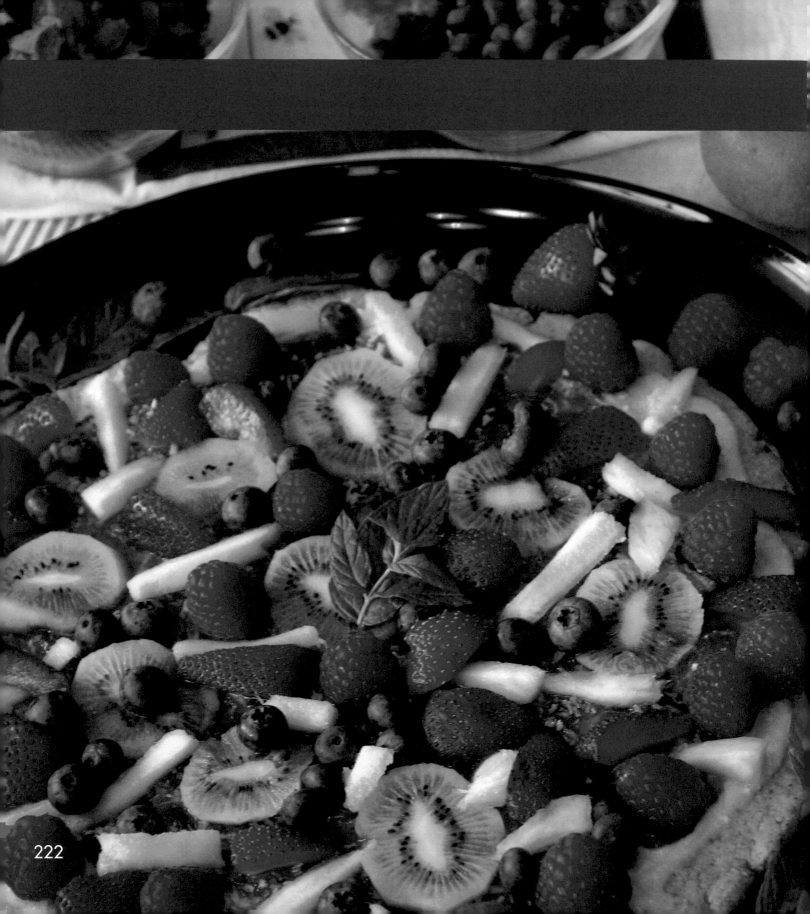

Fruit Pizza

This is hands down the prettiest recipe in the book, in our humble opinion. This is a fun project to make with a gathering of friends or family. Be creative with the way you organize the fruit and enjoy fully. No guilt here. Just plenty of antioxidant rich berries, vitamin C, essential fats, and even fiber. Guests will definitely want you to write down the recipe.

Serves 10

1½ cups whole wheat pastry flour
3 tablespoons flour
½ cup slivered almonds
½ cup walnuts
1 teaspoon baking powder
½ cup oats
¼ teaspoon salt
¼ teaspoon cinnamon
3 tablespoons sugar

4 tablespoons unsalted butter
1 teaspoon vanilla extract
1 medium egg
3 tablespoons lowfat 1% milk
¼ cup lowfat cottage cheese
¼ cup neufchatel cheese (lowfat cream cheese)
½ teaspoon vanilla extract
2 tablespoons agave nectar or honey

Fruit (get creative here and choose your favorite fruits):
1 cup strawberries, rinsed and hulled
1 tablespoon agave nectar or honey
1 tablespoon dried coconut, shredded
2 med kiwi fruit, peeled and thinly sliced
¼ cup raspberries
1 cup sliced mango
¼ cup blueberries
½ cup strawberries

First preheat the oven to 375°F. For the crust you will want to grind the almonds and walnuts in a coffee grinder or food processor so that they resemble flour or have a fine mealy texture. It helps to combine with a tablespoon of flour so that the nuts themselves don't turn into "nut butter" in your coffee grinder. We used one tablespoon flour for the almonds and 2 for the walnuts (and ground them in 2 batches).

Stir together all of the dry ingredients (whole wheat pastry flour through sugar). Add butter, vanilla, egg, and milk and mix on speed 2 until mixture comes together into a ball. Roll out this "cookie crust" like you would a pizza crust. It is helpful to do this on a cookie sheet lined with parchment paper so it is ready to go right into the oven. Shape it into a large round disk that is about ¼ inch thick. Use your hands to soften the edges. Bake crust for about 13 minutes or until slightly golden and cooked in the center. Remove and allow to cool before adding toppings.

Purée cottage cheese, cream cheese, vanilla, and honey in a mixer or blender. Set aside.

On the stovetop or in the microwave, combine 1 cup strawberries with honey (or substitute strawberry jam for the honey). Bring to a simmer for just about 2 minutes. Allow to cool slightly then purée.

Now the fun begins. Spread a thin layer of the creamy mixture atop the cooled crust. Follow this up with the strawberry purée. Sprinkle with a tablespoon of shredded coconut. Now use your imagination to decorate the top with your favorite seasonal fruit. We used kiwi, raspberries, mango, strawberries and blueberries.

Per Serving:
310 Calories;
14g Fat (4g sat);
9g Protein;
39g Carbohydrate;
6g Dietary Fiber;
36mg Cholesterol;
150mg Sodium.

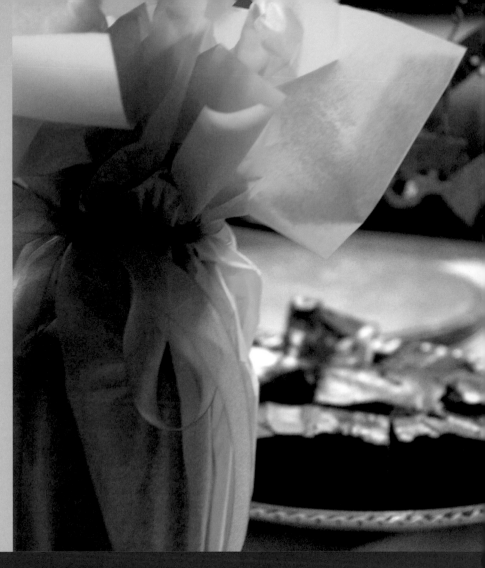

These gluten free brownies are a real cinch to make. They are much chewier than our other brownies and you can experiment with adding miniature chocolate chips or frosting, but we like these very well just the way they are.

Makes about 20 brownies

Gluten Free Brownies

8 tablespoons unsalted butter (1 stick)
½ cup applesauce (or you can use another 7
    tablespoons of butter for really rich brownies)
1½ cups sugar
1 cup plus 2 tablespoons cocoa powder
    (yes, this sounds like a lot of cocoa powder)
½ teaspoon salt
¾ teaspoon vanilla extract
3 large eggs
¾ -1 cup brown rice flour

Preheat oven to 325°F. Line an 8 x 12 nonstick baking dish with parchment paper. Melt butter in microwave or on stovetop. Mix in applesauce if using, sugar, cocoa powder and salt until mixture is smooth. Stir in vanilla extract. Beat in eggs one at a time with a wooden spoon. Stir in flour until it is fully incorporated. Spread mixture evenly into prepared pan. Bake for about 25 minutes. Cool completely on rack before slicing.

Per Serving:
163 Calories;
6g Fat (4g sat);
3g Protein;
27g Carbohydrate;
3g Dietary Fiber;
44mg Cholesterol;
113mg Sodium.

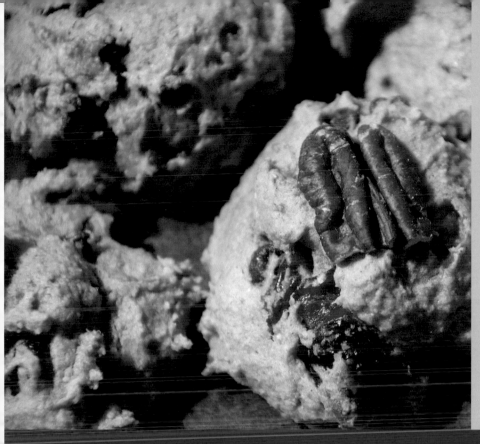

These are out of the ordinary! These are great any time of year but they have always been a big hit during the Fall and as holiday gifts.

Makes 36 cookies

Harvest Cookies

Preheat oven to 375°F. Combine flours, baking powder, baking soda, and spices in a medium bowl. In a large bowl, beat butter and sugar until creamy and fluffy. Beat in pumpkin, apple butter, egg, and vanilla. Gradually add flour mixture to pumpkin mixture. Beat at low speed until well blended. Stir in cranberries and chocolate chips. Drop dough by heaping tablespoons onto ungreased cookie sheet. Press ½ pecan into the top of each cookie.

Bake 10 to 12 minutes or until golden. Let cookies stand on cookie sheet for about a minute and then transfer to wire racks to cool.

Per Cookie:
93 Calories;
5g Fat (2g sat);
1g Protein;
13g Carbohydrate;
1g Dietary Fiber,
12mg Cholesterol;
60mg Sodium.

1 cup whole wheat pastry flour
1 cup all purpose unbleached flour
1 teaspoon baking powder
½ teaspoon baking soda
1 teaspoon cinnamon
½ teaspoon allspice
½ cup butter, softened (or non-hydrogenated vegetable spread or shortening)
½ cup sugar
1 cup canned pumpkin
½ cup apple butter
1 medium egg
1 teaspoon vanilla
¾ cup dried cranberries
½ cup semisweet (miniature) chocolate chips
36 pecan halves

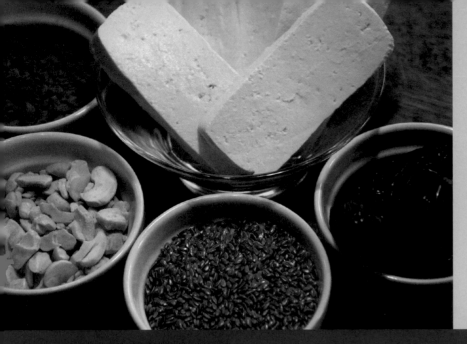

Talk about a sneaky way to make a heart-healthy dessert look more like an over-the-top indulgence. You'll have to convince your guests and yourself that you're actually eating something relatively good for you with heart-healthy phytosterols, antioxidants, and fiber!

Serves 10

Happy Heart Cake

Preheat oven to 350°F. Grease two 8X8 cake pans (or one 13½ X 9 inch baking dish) and coat lightly with flour. In a large bowl mix first 4 ingredients. Grind flax seeds to a fine powder in a blender. Add ½ cup water to blender and process until thick and frothy. Add dates and soaking liquid, tofu, maple syrup, applesauce, oil and extract. Blend again until smooth. Transfer to a large bowl. Blend dry ingredients into the wet. Divide batter evenly between pans. Bake 20 to 25 minutes. Cool for at least 10 minutes on wire rack then invert cake onto wire racks and allow to cool completely.

Make frosting while cake is cooling. Melt chocolate in double boiler or over low heat, stirring until smooth. Grind cashews in blender. Add ⅓ cup water, tofu, maple syrup and vanilla and blend until smooth. Add melted chocolate and blend again. Transfer to medium bowl and refrigerate until chilled. Frost one layer at a time, spreading about ⅔ cup frosting over top of one layer. Place second layer on top of frosted layer and frost top and sides of cake.

Per Serving:
339 Calories;
14g Fat (5g sat);
8g Protein;
54g Carbohydrate;
7g Dietary Fiber;
0mg Cholesterol;
287mg Sodium.

1½ cups whole wheat flour
¾ cup unsweetened cocoa powder
1 tablespoon baking powder
1 teaspoon baking soda
2 tablespoons flax seeds
½ cup pitted dates, soaked in 1 cup hot water for 30 minutes
6 ounces firm silken tofu
½ cup maple syrup
½ cup applesauce
2 teaspoons canola oil
1½ teaspoons vanilla or almond extract

Frosting
1 cup semisweet chocolate chips
½ cup raw cashews
6 ounces extra firm silken tofu
2 tablespoons maple syrup
1 teaspoon vanilla extract

226

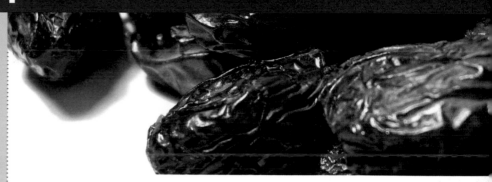

Maple Date Bars

We've mentioned before our fondness for dates (and maple syrup) – so of course they are going to appear in one of our more decadent desserts. The richness of the nuts, the nut butter and the butter is what makes these bars more of a splurge, but they are still loaded with plenty of goodness so you shouldn't feel one bit guilty before, during, or after eating these. Sixteen slices make these bars fairly small, which is also why they make a healthy indulgence, weighing in under 200 calories. Enjoy the sweetness.

Makes 16 bars

1 cup apple juice
1½ cups pitted dates
½ teaspoon maple extract
½ teaspoon vanilla extract
½ cup water
1½ cups whole wheat pastry flour
½ cup walnuts
1 cup rolled oats
1½ teaspoons ground cinnamon
¼ teaspoon baking powder
¼ teaspoon baking soda
½ teaspoon sea salt
4 tablespoons butter
2 tablespoons almond butter
¼ cup maple syrup

Preheat oven to 350°F. Lightly coat a 8x8-inch baking pan with cooking spray and line with parchment paper. Bring 1 cup of apple juice to simmer in a medium saucepan. Add dates; simmer until very soft and thick, whisking and stirring occasionally, about 10 minutes. Cool to room temperature. Stir in maple and vanilla extracts.

Combine flour, oats, walnuts, cinnamon, baking powder, baking soda, and salt in the bowl of a food processor filled with steel S-blade. Process or pulse on low setting until well mixed and walnuts are finely chopped. Add butter, almond butter and maple syrup and process again until combined. Mixture will appear like thick cookie batter.

Press half of oat mixture evenly over bottom of prepared baking pan.

Blend date mixture in a blender until smooth, adding additional water if necessary. You can also do this step in a food processor. Spread date mixture over the first layer of oat mixture in the pan. Cover the date layer with remaining oat mixture, pressing gently to adhere.

Bake about 30 to 40 minutes, until brown at edges and golden brown and set in the center. Cool completely in pan on a wire rack. Cut into bars when cool.

Per Serving:
189 Calories;
7g Fat (2g sat);
4g Protein;
30g Carbohydrate;
4g Dietary Fiber;
8mg Cholesterol;
105mg Sodium.

Second only to carrot cake, pumpkin pie is one of the most oft' requested desserts in the Rouse house. It is Dakota's favorite treat – served with a generous portion of our favorite whipped cream, of course. We make the crust using gluten-free ginger snaps and brown rice flour – and you could easily substitute a more traditional crust if desired – however, we love the combination of the ginger and pumpkin, so we love this version!

Serves 8

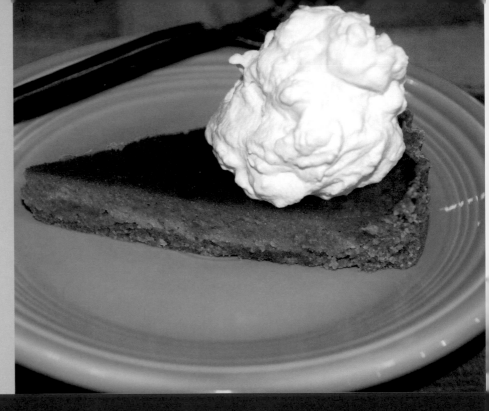

Ginger Crust Pumpkin Pie

Crust:
1½ cups ginger snaps, crushed
¾ cup brown rice flour
1 tbsp brown sugar
5 tablespoons butter

Filling:
1 can pumpkin (16 ounce)
2 eggs
¼ cup maple syrup
1 teaspoon ground cinnamon
½ teaspoon salt
½ teaspoon ground ginger
⅛ teaspoon ground nutmeg
1½ cups milk of choice milk (soy, lowfat cow's, goat's) plus 1 teaspoon vanilla extract (alternatively you can use sweetened condensed milk for a much sweeter version of this pie).

In the bowl of a food processor fitted with S blade, combine ingredients for crust. Pulse until well combined and then press into a 9-inch pie plate coated with cooking oil spray. Chill about thirty minutes.

After the crust has chilled, preheat the oven to 375°F.

In a medium size mixing bowl, whisk pumpkin and eggs together. Gradually add maple syrup, cinnamon, salt, ginger, and nutmeg. Stir in milk (and vanilla if using regular milk).

Pour pumpkin mixture into prepared pie shell. Cover edge of pie with foil. Bake in preheated oven for 30 minutes. Remove foil and return the pie to the oven. Bake for an additional 10 or 15 minutes or until the center appears set when lightly touched. Cool on a wire rack. Cover and chill to store.

Per Serving:
344 Calories;
13g Fat (5g sat);
7g Protein;
52g Carbohydrate;
2g Dietary Fiber;
21mg Cholesterol;
354mg Sodium.

228

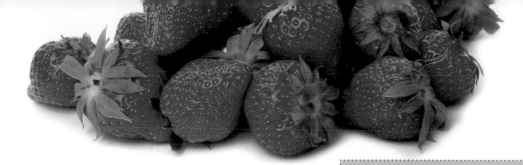

Preheat oven to 375°F. Coat a baking sheet with cooking oil spray. Combine oats, flour, sucanat, cinnamon, and baking soda in medium size bowl. Stir until blended. Stir in oil and 2 tablespoons yogurt to make a soft, somewhat sticky dough. Add remaining yogurt if dough is too stiff.

Place dough on the prepared baking sheet and pat into a 10" circle. Place a 9" cake pan on the dough and trace around it with a sharp knife. With fingers push up and pinch the dough around the outside of the circle to make a 9" circle with a rim ¼ " high. Bake for 15 minutes, or until firm and golden. Remove from oven and set aside to cool. With a spatula, gently ease the crust onto large, flat serving plate.

Wash the strawberries and pat dry. Slice off stems. In a small microwaveable bowl or on the stovetop, combine strawberry spread and vanilla. Microwave on high power for 15 seconds or until melted.

Brush or dab a generous tablespoon of the heated strawberry spread evenly over the crust. Arrange the strawberries, cut side down, evenly over the crust. Brush or dab the remaining spread evenly over the strawberries, making sure that you get some of the spread between the strawberries to secure them.

Refrigerate for at least 30 minutes, or until the spread has jelled. Cut into wedges.

Per Serving:
108 Calories;
3g Fat (trace sat);
2g Protein;
18g Carbohydrate;
2g Dietary Fiber;
Trace Cholesterol;
38mg Sodium.

The crust on this tart is wonderful and simple to make. It is always a hit at our house. It's a little bit like the miniature, scaled-down version of the fruit pizza and a great use of all those extra summer strawberries. Antioxidants (anthocyanins) in strawberries have been shown to support the heart, the eyes, and may have anti-inflammatory effects in the body. Strawberries are loaded with vitamins and fiber too!

Serves 10

Oat-Cinnamon Crust
⅔ cup rolled oats
½ cup unbleached organic flour
1 tablespoon sucanat or organic sugar
1 teaspoon cinnamon
¼ teaspoon baking soda
2 tablespoons canola oil
2 to 3 tablespoons nonfat plain yogurt

Strawberry Filling
1½ pints strawberries
¼ cup all-fruit strawberry spread
½ teaspoon vanilla

Strawberry Tart

Palate Pleaser Sorbet

Combine water and sugar in a small saucepan on the stove and heat until the sugar is dissolved. Refrigerate until cool.

Place watermelon in a blender in small batches (blender about half full). Add a little bit of the sugar water to facilitate the blending. Purée well and then strain into container for ice cream maker or a freezer-proof bowl. Continue this process until all of the watermelon has been puréed.

Do the same with the raspberries. Use a mesh strainer to prevent the raspberry seeds from getting into the sorbet. Combine the raspberry purée with the watermelon purée and add the fresh lime juice. Stir well to combine. If you are using an ice-cream maker then you can go ahead and follow the manufacturer's instructions for freezing at this point. If you are using a freezer alone, freeze the mixture for about a half hour at a time, stirring in between until desired consistency is obtained. The sorbet is best served as fresh as possible.

Notes: Individuals with "sugar issues" may omit the sugar. The sorbet will be slightly more bitter due to the raspberries and lime juice. You may also vary the amounts of the fruits and if you have a lot more watermelon to use then go ahead and add it!!

A very refreshing and tart treat. Watermelon is a good source of vitamins C, B6, B1, potassium, magnesium, and beta-carotene. Watermelon also contains a concentrated source of lycopene, which has been found to be protective against certain cancers.

Serves 8

½ cup water
¼ cup sugar
10 cups seedless watermelon, chopped
1 pint raspberries
juice from one lime
ice

Per Serving:
135 Calories;
1g Fat (0 sat);
2g Protein;
32g Carbohydrate;
4g Dietary Fiber;
0mg Cholesterol;
6mg Sodium.

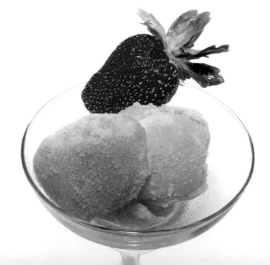

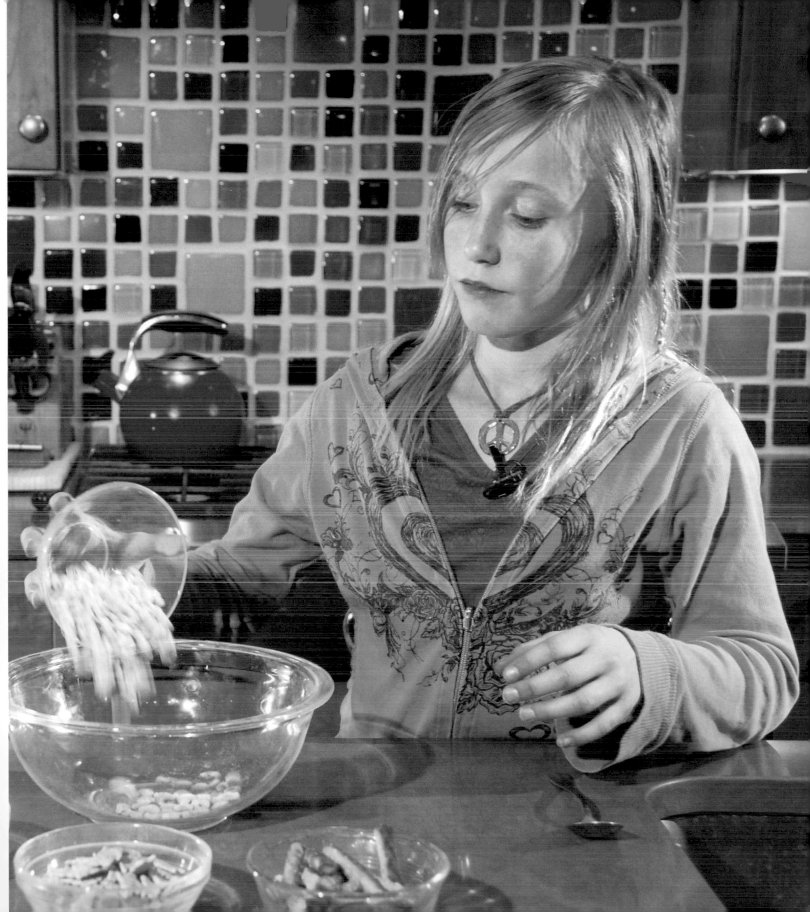

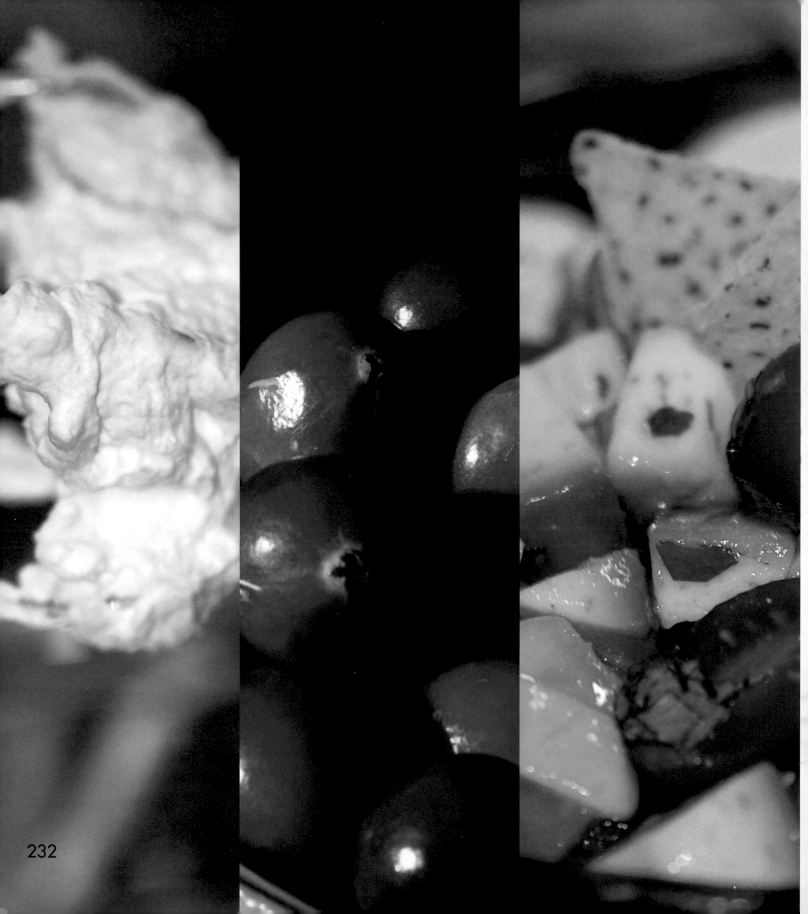

Nothing would be more tiresome than eating and drinking if God had not made them a pleasure as well as a necessity. ~Voltaire

Essentials

Everyone needs their "go to" dressing or special sauce that they know is tasty and reliable. For us, it's the Divine Dressing (p. 82). We use it to marinate poultry and fish and we use it on almost every salad we make. Sometimes we add more ginger and sometimes we'll substitute garlic – but the base is there and it's our fail-safe.

We are also big on salsas, which we feel accentuate the positive in most entrees. The salsas here are perfect for parties or potlucks – they are both aesthetically pleasing and super tasty.

Almond Butter Dressing

This dressing has a bit of a Thai flare to it. It is wonderful on top of grilled poultry, tofu, or tempeh and also wonderful to serve on the side of stir fries and rice dishes. You can also use it as a dipping dressing for vegetables.

Makes 1½ cups

½ cup tofu
3 tablespoons almond butter
2 tablespoons wheat-free tamari soy sauce
4 tablespoons rice vinegar
2 tablespoons agave nectar (or honey)
1½ tablespoons fresh ginger, peeled and minced
4 tablespoons light coconut milk
1 scallion, finely minced

Combine all the ingredients in a blender and blend until smooth and creamy.

Per Serving
(2 tablespoons):
46 Calories; 3g Fat
(trace sat.); 2g Protein;
4g Carbohydrate;
trace Dietary Fiber;
0mg Cholesterol;
170mg Sodium.

Apple Cinnamon Dressing

Bring apple juice, sherry, cinnamon, and allspice to a boil. Continue to reduce over medium heat until mixture is about ¼ cup. Strain mixture into canola oil and whisk until emulsified together. Allow mixture to come to room temperature.

Per Serving:
(2 tablespoons):
33 Calories; 3g Fat
(trace sat.); trace Protein;
1g Carbohydrate;
trace Dietary Fiber;
0mg Cholesterol;
trace Sodium.

This is a very autumn-inspired dressing. It is perfect served along side pork. It is also nice on top of a fresh spinach salad where you can pour it over the spinach while it is still warm and add a bit of freshly cooked and chopped bacon.

Makes 2 cups

2 cups unsweetened apple juice
1 tablespoon sherry
1 tablespoon cinnamon
1 teaspoon allspice
¼ cup canola or olive oil

Rocky Mountain Biscuits

Preheat the oven to 425°F. Cover a baking sheet with a piece of parchment paper.

Whisk together the flour, baking powder, and salt together into a large bowl. Using two knives or a pastry blender, cut in the butter until the texture ranges from cornmeal to the size of small peas. (These two steps can be done quickly in a food processor.) Using a fork, gradually mix in the yogurt, then the milk, until the dough is quite soft and somewhat sticky. Work quickly without overworking the dough. Turn it out onto a lightly floured surface and knead it briefly, just long enough to get it to hold together. Roll it out so it is about 1¼ inches thick, and cut it into 2 inch rounds. Arrange the biscuits on the prepared baking sheet, and bake in the center of the oven until they are deep golden, puffed and cooked through, 18 to 20 minutes.

Makes 10-12

1½ cups whole wheat pastry flour
2 teaspoons baking powder
1 teaspoon salt
4 tablespoons unsalted butter, chilled
⅓ cup nonfat Greek-style yogurt
½ cup lowfat buttermilk

Per Serving:
116 Calories;
5g Fat (3g sat);
3g Protein;
15g Carbohydrate;
2g Dietary Fiber;
13mg Cholesterol;
327mg Sodium.

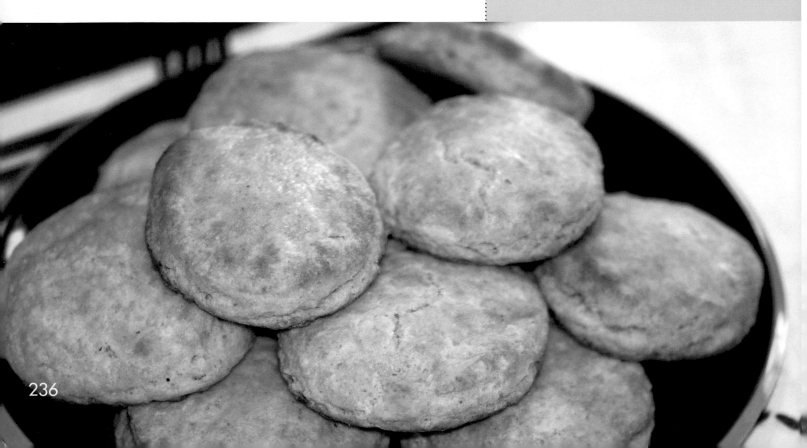

236

Black Bean Salsa

This black bean salsa adds a Caribbean flair in addition to heart-healthy fiber and vitamin C. Enjoy!

Serves 6

2 cups cooked black beans
1 medium mango, peeled and chopped (about 1 cup)
1 medium red bell pepper, chopped (about ½ cup)
⅓ cup sliced green onions (2 to 3 medium)
2 tablespoons orange juice
1 tablespoon rice wine vinegar
2 teaspoons lime juice

Toss all ingredients together. Refrigerate until ready to serve.

Per Serving
(about ½ cup):
108 Calories; trace Fat
(trace sat); 6g Protein;
22g Carbohydrate; 6g Dietary
Fiber; 0mg Cholesterol;
3mg Sodium.

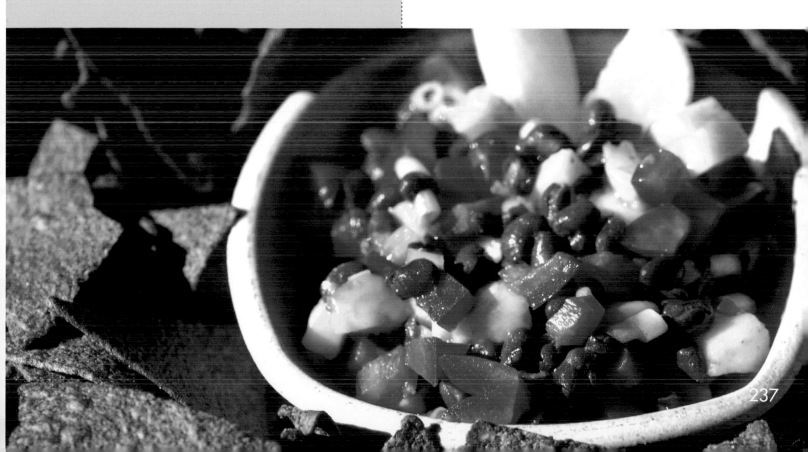

Chantilly

Chantilly is a sweetened whipped cream – it is also the name of a town in France where whipped cream is rumored to have been invented. Debra loves whipped cream so much that on a trip to France in 2005 she made a special trip to Chantilly with Dakota and Elli, just so they could eat whipped cream in the gardens of the very castle where this luscious cream was born. To us, the best dessert hands down is fresh berries with homemade whipped cream. We always chose organic whipping cream to make sure we are getting hormone- and pesticide-free cream. Here is our basic recipe. Sometimes we'll substitute cinnamon-sugar in place of the agave and vanilla or we'll use maple syrup and extract (this is great on pumpkin pie).

32 servings

1 pint whipped cream
2 teaspoons agave nectar
½ teaspoon vanilla extract

Beat all the ingredients together in a large bowl. It may help to chill the bowl and the beaters ahead of time. It usually takes at least 5 minutes of beating/whipping to achieve desired fluffy consistency. Be careful not to overwhip or you'll end up with butter.

Per Serving:
54 Calories;
6g Fat (3g sat);
trace Protein;
1g Carbohydrate;
0g Dietary Fiber;
20mg Cholesterol;
6mg Sodium.

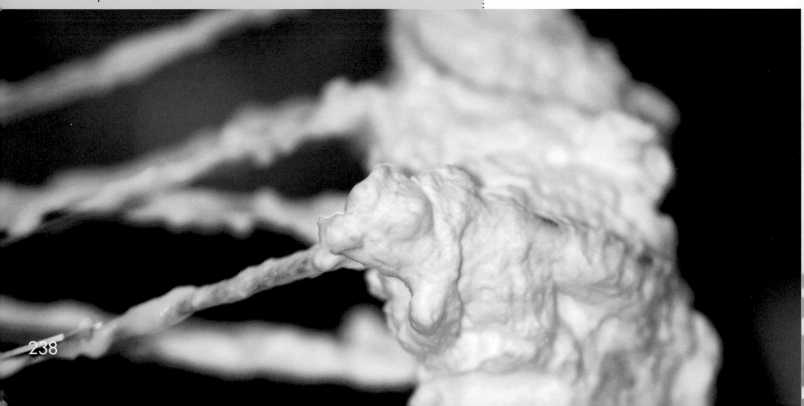

Cranberry Salsa

Combine cranberries, sugar, onions, cilantro, lime juice, rind, ginger root and jalapeño pepper in food processor bowl. Pulse on/off until mixture is chopped (not puréed). Stir in sour cream if desired. Cover and chill at least 2 hours or up to 1 week.

Per Serving (about ½ cup): 108 Calories; trace Fat (trace sat); 6g Protein; 22g Carbohydrate; 6g Dietary Fiber; 0mg Cholesterol; 3mg Sodium.

This is another salsa that is delicious served with pork, turkey, or chicken. It is a surprising and spicy addition to the Thanksgiving buffet.

Makes 2 cups

1 cup fresh cranberries
⅓ cup sugar
2 green onions chopped
¼ cup fresh cilantro
1 lime, grated and juiced
2 teaspoons minced ginger root
½ to 1 whole small jalapeño pepper, seeds removed and diced
*   (start with ½ pepper then adjust for desired spicyness)*
2 tablespoons lowfat sour cream or plain yogurt, (optional)

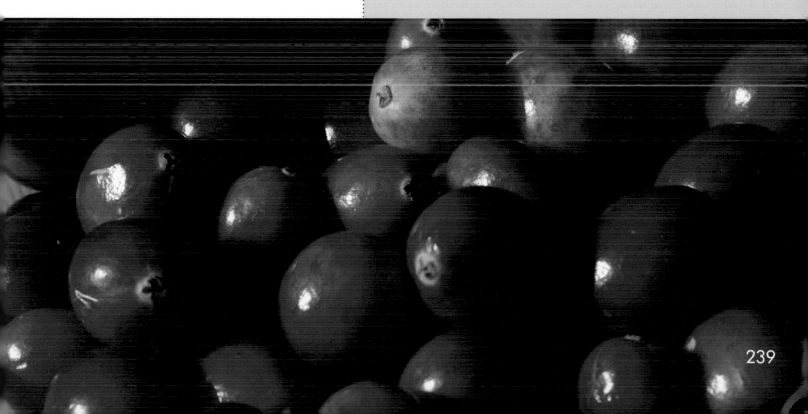

Creamy Watercress Dressing

Whisk together the yogurt, mayonnaise, watercress, green onions, lemon juice and peel. Refrigerate until ready to use.

Per Serving
22 Calories; 2g Fat
(trace sat); Protein;
1g Carbohydrate; trace
Dietary Fiber;
2mg Cholesterol;
17mg Sodium

This dressing is delicious on top of baby lettuces, fresh tomatoes, cooked beets, and on top of poultry and meat dishes.

Makes 1½ cups – 24 servings

¾ cup plain yogurt
¼ cup mayonnaise
¼ cup fresh watercress, chopped
2 green onions, chopped
1 tablespoon fresh lemon juice
2 teaspoons grated lemon peel

Watercress is a member of the mustard (Cruciferae) family. It is an excellent source of phytochemicals (antioxidants), known as isothiocyanates. The particular isothiocyanate found in watercress is called phenyl ethyl isothiocyanate (PEITC). It has been linked to a decreased risk of certain cancers including lung cancer. A recent study done by researchers at the University of Ulster in England showed that eating watercress may reduce damage to DNA and lower cancer risk.

In the study, researchers found that in a group of sixty (cancer-free) adults (half of them were smokers), those who ate approximately 3 ounces of watercress daily for 8 weeks in addition to their normal diets had higher levels of antioxidants and fewer DNA damaging chemicals in their blood.

Although this was a rather short term study in terms of long term cancer protection and prevention, it does give good reason to go ahead and add a little watercress to your diet. Watercress also provides a healthy dose of beta carotene, vitamin C, fiber, and potassium.

Look for watercress with bright green, non-wilting leaves. Use it within a few days of purchase and keep it from getting crushed by other fruits and veggies in the crisper. Try watercress on sandwiches, in salads, tossed with fruits in a fruit salad, stirred into potato or egg salad or blended with cottage cheese for a nice dip or spread. You can also try it cooked in soups, stir fries, scrambled eggs – be creative. Note: the British study was done with raw (uncooked) watercress.

Flaxseed Oil and Lemon Dressing

Refreshingly tart – you may want to adjust the amount of lemon juice and flax seed oil until you get the perfect balance for your palate. We've been making this dressing for years and have adapted it for our taste buds and invite you to do the same.

Makes 1 cup

1 bunch of fresh basil (about 1/4 cup), chopped (or 2 teaspoons dried)
2 cloves garlic, finely minced
¼ cup lemon juice
¼ cup flaxseed oil
¼ cup olive oil
1 tablespoon wheat-free tamari soy sauce or Bragg's Liquid Aminos
1 teaspoon pure maple syrup
¼ cup water

Wash and dry basil leaves. Chop garlic cloves and basil then add to a blender with the liquids and blend to a creamy consistency. You may add 1 to 2 tablespoons of this to a serving of steamed rice, salad, or vegetable of your choice as a dressing.

Per Serving
32 Calories;
3g Fat (trace sat);
trace Protein;
1g Carbohydrate;
trace Dietary Fiber;
0mg Cholesterol;
trace Sodium

Flaxseeds are full of alpha linolenic acid (ALA), an omega-3 fat that the body can convert to eicosapentaenoic acid (EPA), the same omega-3 fat found in fish like salmon. This conversion relies on the presence and activity of an enzyme known as delta-6 desaturase, which may be inhibited in individuals with diabetes and/or with the consumption of saturated fat and alcohol. Studies have shown that omega-3 fats from flaxseed oil may help control high blood pressure, protect against heart disease, certain cancers, and type 2 diabetes, have a positive effect on bone health, and help reduce high cholesterol. Flaxseed oil is a more concentrated source of ALA than the flaxseeds themselves, so vegetarians or individuals who do not eat fish may want to consider adding flaxseed oil as a staple to their diets.

Gluten/Dairy Free Pizza Crust

In a small bowl, dissolve the yeast in half of the warm water, add sugar (or agave) and mix well. Set aside for 15 minutes. Preheat the oven to 425°F. Lightly oil a large pizza pan or cookie sheet. Prepare the toppings for the pizza (tomato paste or sauce, veggies, cheese, etc).

Stir together the dry ingredients (brown rice flour through corn meal) in a large mixing bowl (or stand up mixer). Add the yeast mixture and mix well, adding the remaining water and olive oil a little at a time until the dough is fairly thick and sticky. Place the dough on a clean surface coated with a little bit of additional brown rice flour. Knead the dough for about a minute. Place the dough in the middle of the prepared pan and spread it around (or roll out) evenly. Bake on the top rack of the oven for about 5 minutes until the dough has lightly set. Remove from the oven and reduce the oven temperature to 375°F.

Add the toppings of your choice to the pizza. Return to the oven and continue to bake for an additional 12 to 15 minutes.

Makes 1 large crust (approximately 4 servings)

½ teaspoon active dry yeast
1 cup warm water, divided
1 teaspoon sugar, agave nectar or honey
1 cup brown rice flour
3 tablespoons potato flour
¼ cup amaranth flour
1 tablespoon ground flax seed
1 tablespoon yellow cornmeal
1 tablespoon olive oil

Per Serving
(crust only):
291 Calories; 7g Fat
(1g sat); 7g Protein;
51g Carbohydrate;
5g Dietary Fiber;
0mg Cholesterol;
13mg Sodium.

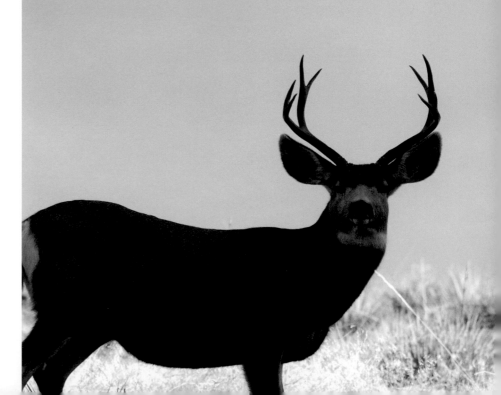

242

Jalapeño Lime Butter

8 servings

4 tablespoons unsalted butter, softened
½ small jalapeno pepper, seeded and minced
½ teaspoon grated lime rind
1 teaspoon fresh cilantro, finely chopped

Per Serving (½
tablespoon):
51 Calories; 6g Fat
(4g sat); trace Protein; trace
Carbohydrate; trace Dietary
Fiber; 16mg Cholesterol;
1mg Sodium.

Combine softened butter with jalapeno, lime zest and cilantro in a small bowl. Mix together with a fork. Once the ingredients are well-mixed then place the mound of butter in the middle of a sheet of plastic wrap and roll it into a log shape. Refrigerate the log at least 30 minutes or until ready to use. It is delicious on top of Our Favorite Salmon (p. 173) or even on top of brown rice with veggies.

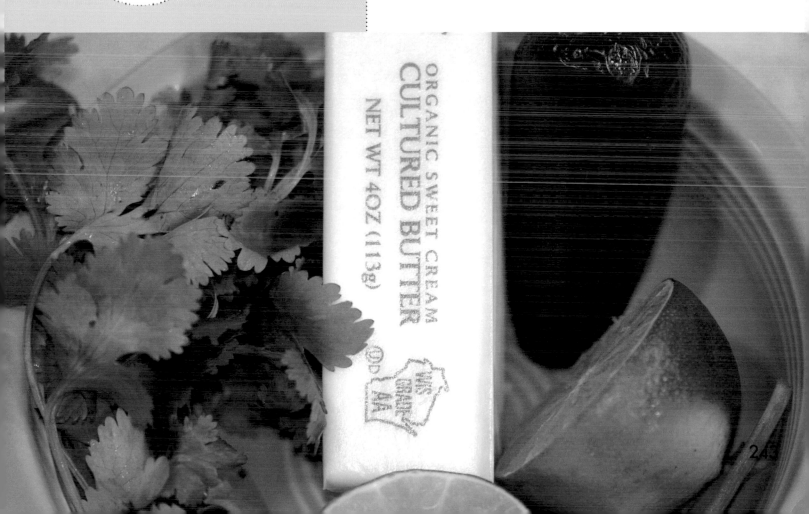

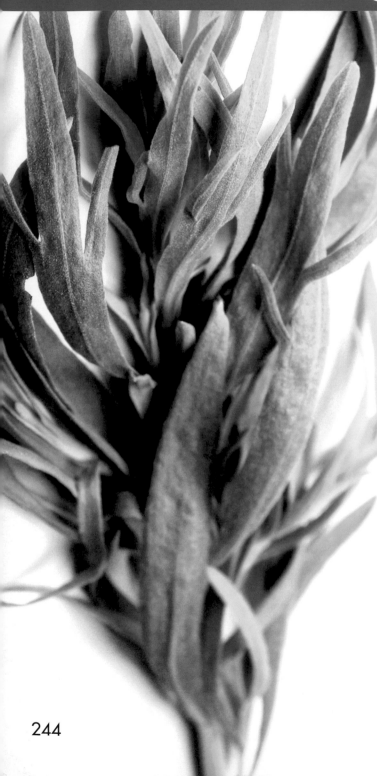

Lemon Tarragon Vinaigrette

Tarragon is used a lot in French cooking. It also has use as a medicinal herb. Ancient Greeks chewed tarragon leaves to ease the pain of toothaches since tarragon has a numbing quality. Tarragon has also been used to aid digestion and offers healing properties for stomach cramps. Tarragon also has mild sedative qualities – so you may want to save this vinaigrette for evening meals!

Makes 1½ cups

2 tablespoons chopped fresh tarragon leaves
2 tablespoons Dijon mustard
1 tablespoon minced shallot
1½ teaspoons sea salt
½ teaspoon lemon pepper or ¾ teaspoon ground
*   black pepper*
½ cup extra virgin olive oil
¼ cup canola oil
½ cup white wine vinegar
1 tablespoon fresh lemon juice

In a small bowl, whisk together tarragon, mustard, shallots, sea salt, lemon pepper, oils, vinegar and lemon juice. Refrigerate until ready to use and whisk again just before serving.

Per Serving
(62 Calories;
7g Fat (1g sat);
trace Protein;
1g Carbohydrate; trace
Dietary Fiber;
0mg Cholesterol;
140mg Sodium

Mango-Avocado Salsa

This salsa is loaded with vitamin C. Mangoes are also a great source of beta-carotene and fiber. Avocados provide heart healthy monounsaturated fat as well as glutathione, which is a powerful antioxidant. Cilantro is a natural detoxifier.

Serves 4

1 avocado, peeled, pitted and chopped
1 mango, peeled, pitted and chopped
1 tablespoon fresh cilantro, minced
1 cup cherry tomatoes, halved
2 tablespoons lime juice
½ teaspoon sea salt
1 jalapeno pepper, seeded and minced

Lightly toss all ingredients together in a nonmetal bowl. Refrigerate until ready to serve.

Per Serving
126 Calories;
8g Fat (1g sat);
2g Protein;
15g Carbohydrate;
3g Dietary Fiber;
0mg Cholesterol;
245mg Sodium

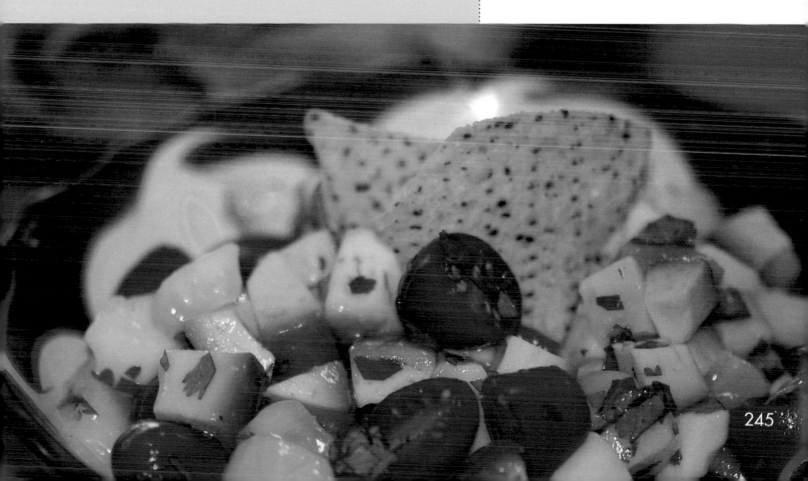

245

Pesto

The great thing about pesto is you can spread it on or add to it just about everything and anything. You can substitute other greens for the basil. We like to make cilantro pesto every once in a while.

Makes 3 ½ cups

2 ½ cups firmly packed fresh basil leaves
1 cup olive oil
¼ cup pine nuts
¼ cup walnuts, or almonds
3 cloves garlic, or more as desired
salt and pepper, to taste

Place all ingredients in blender or food processor. Cover and blend on medium speed about 3 minutes, until smooth, stopping occasionally to scrape sides. Delicious tossed with hot cooked pasta.

Per Serving
(2 Tablespoons):
72 Calories; 8g Fat
(1g sat); 1g Protein;
trace Carbohydrate;
trace Dietary Fiber;
0mg Cholesterol;
trace Sodium

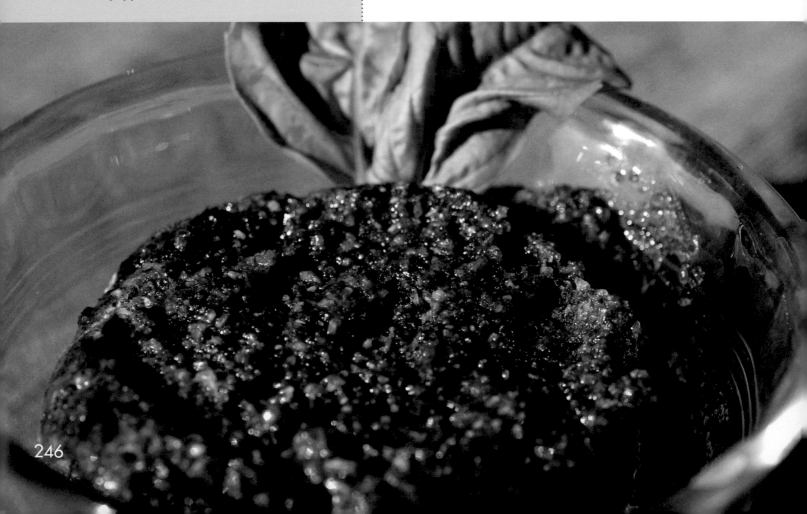

Raspberry Peach Sauce

Place raspberries, peach slices, juice and maple syrup in blender or food processor. Cover and blend on high speed about 1 minute or until smooth. Heat blended mixture in saucepan until hot; reduce heat. Keep warm. This is wonderful on top of yogurt, vanilla or ginger ice cream or frozen yogurt.

Per Serving
58 Calories; trace
Fat (trace sat); trace
Protein; 15g Carbohydrate;
2g Dietary Fiber;
0mg Cholesterol;
1mg Sodium.

This sauce epitomizes the freshness of summer – however the availability of frozen fruit year-round makes it possible to enjoy this scrumptious sauce anytime.

Serves 4

½ cup raspberries
2 medium peaches, peeled and sliced
2 tablespoons apple juice
2 tablespoons maple syrup

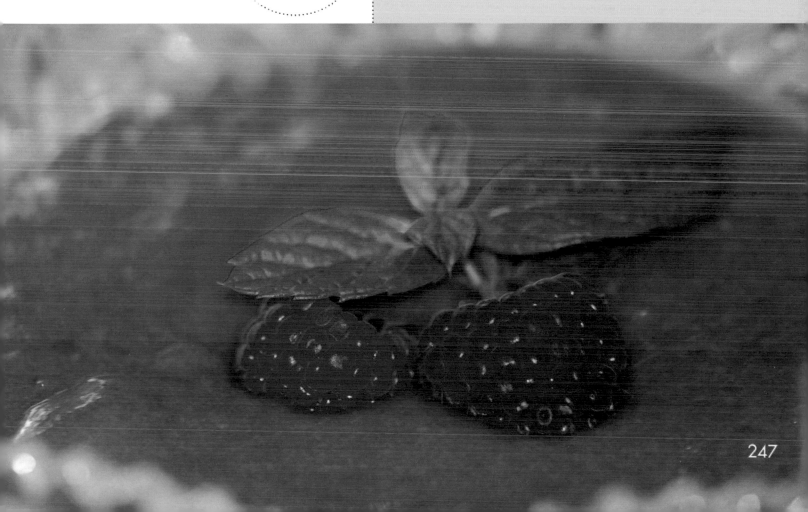

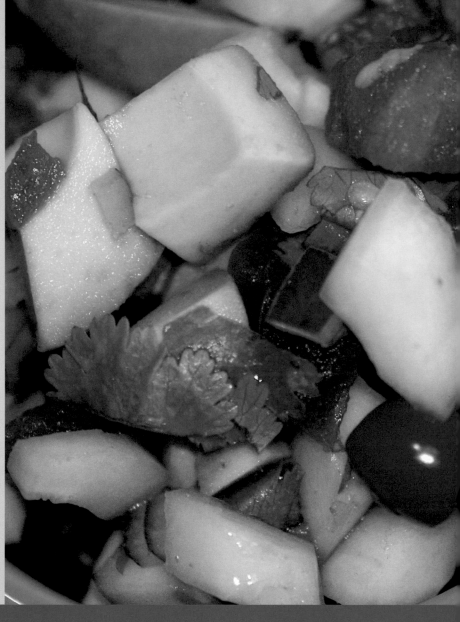

This "salsa" is great on top of fish. It can also be eaten as is, like a watermelon gazpacho. The cooling sweetness of the watermelon collides with the fiery spice of the jalapeno for a real flavor rush. Watermelon is packed with antioxidant vitamins and lycopene, which has been studied for its antioxidant and anticancer benefits. Watermelon is also a surprisingly decent source of magnesium and B vitamins.

Serves 2 to 4

Red, White, and Green Salsa

2 cups watermelon, seeded and cubed
1 cup jicama, peeled and diced
1 medium celery stalk, chopped
½ cup avocado, diced
¼ cup fresh cilantro, chopped
1 to 2 tablespoons jalapeno chile pepper, diced
2 tablespoons fresh lime juice
¼ teaspoon sea salt

Mix all ingredients in nonmetal bowl. Adjust amount of jalapeno according to your personal "heat" tolerance. Cover and refrigerate at least 1 hour to blend flavors but no longer than 2 days. Stir salsa before serving.

Per Serving:
40 Calories; trace Fat
(7.8% calories from fat);
1g Protein;
9g Carbohydrate;
2g Dietary Fiber;
0mg Cholesterol;
130mg Sodium.

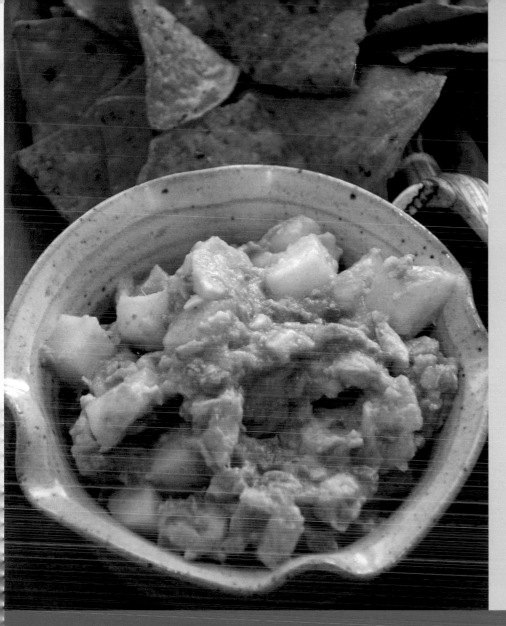

Blending the best of both worlds here – Mexico and Hawaii. It is very difficult to eat this and not feel like you're that much closer to the beach!

Serves 4

Pineapple Guacamole

Combine avocado, lime juice, salsa, jalapeno, salt and pepper and mash together with a fork. Stir in diced pineapple.

Per Serving:
103 Calories; 8g Fat
(1g sat); 1g Protein;
9g Carbohydrate;
2g Dietary Fiber;
0mg Cholesterol;
85mg Sodium.

1 avocado
1 tablespoon lime juice
2 tablespoons salsa
1 teaspoon jalapeno chile pepper, diced
1 dash salt and pepper
1 cup diced pineapple

249

Spicy Peanut Dressing

Place all ingredients in blender or food processor. Cover and blend on medium speed about 3 minutes, or until smooth, stopping occasionally to scrape sides.

Per Serving
48 Calories;
4g Fat (trace sat);
1g Protein;
3g Carbohydrate;
trace Dietary Fiber;
0mg Cholesterol;
67mg Sodium

This dressing is a bit lighter than the Almond Butter Dressing (p. 235). We like to use it in salads and find that it works well on top of mixed greens and grilled chicken breast.

Makes 1¼ cup

¼ *cup natural peanut butter*
2 tablespoons ginger, minced
1 teaspoon chili paste
2 tablespoons low sodium soy sauce
2 tablespoons honey
3 tablespoons rice vinegar
3 tablespoons sesame oil
3 tablespoons low sodium chicken broth, or water

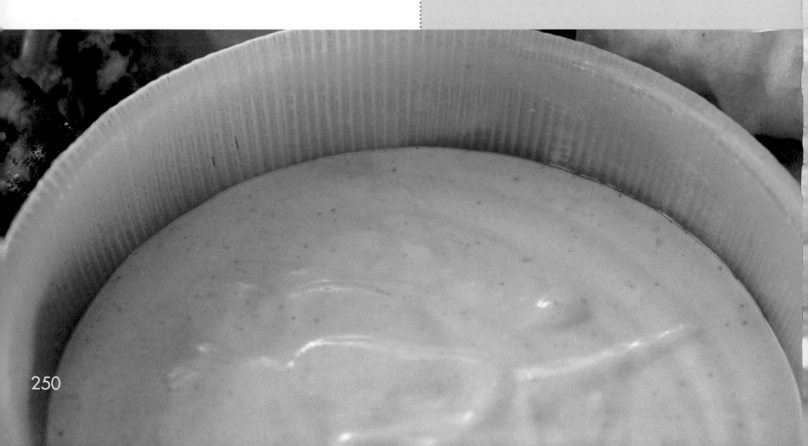

Tomatillo Sauce

Tomatillos look like little green tomatoes enclosed in a husk. They are technically a fruit and are quite popular in Mexico and South American countries. Tomatillos are rich in antioxidant vitamins C and A and contain potassium and folic acid as well.

Serves 6

1 pound fresh tomatillos
2 cloves garlic, peeled and chopped in half
1 jalapeño pepper, seeded and diced
1 cup diced green chiles (drained)
2 tablespoons cilantro leaves
2 tablespoons chopped onion
1 cup diced tomatoes (drained)
1 tablespoon honey
¼ teaspoon salt

Remove husk from tomatillos, rinse and chop. Place in saucepan, cover with water and simmer until tender, about 5 to 7 minutes; drain and discard liquid.

Add tomatillos, garlic, jalapeno pepper, green chili, cilantro, onion, tomatoes, honey, and salt to a food processor and purée.

Serve on top of enchiladas, tacos, or as a dip for tortilla chips

Per Serving:
45 Calories; 1g Fat
(0g sat); 1g Protein;
9g Carbohydrate;
2g Dietary Fiber;
0mg Cholesterol;
96mg Sodium.

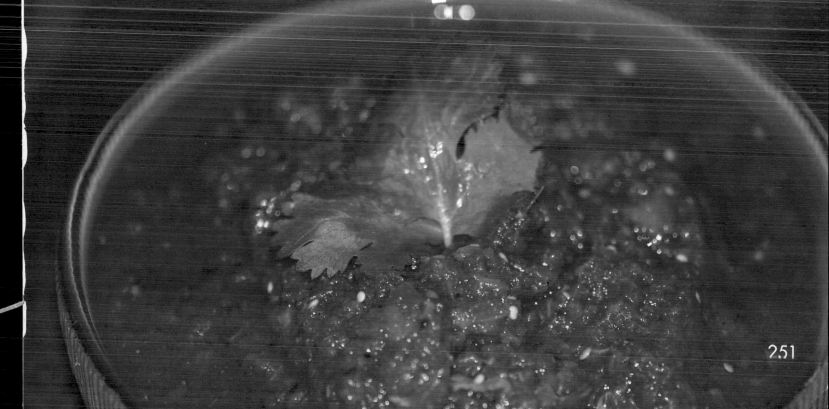

Measurement Conversion

Equivalent Measures

3 teaspoons = 1 tablespoon

4 tablespoons = ¼ cup

5 tablespoons + 1 teaspoon = ⅓ cup

8 tablespoons = ½ cup

12 tablespoons = ¾ cup

16 tablespoons = 1 cup (8 ounces)

2 cups = 1 pint (16 ounces)

4 cups (2 pints) = 1 quart (32 ounces)

8 cups (4 pints) = ½ gallon (64 ounces)

4 quarts = 1 gallon (128 ounces)

Metric Conversion Table

¼ teaspoon = 1 mL

½ teaspoon = 2 mL

1 teaspoon = 5 mL

1 tablespoon = 15 mL

¼ cup = 50 mL

1/3 cup = 75 mL

½ cup = 125 mL

2/3 cup = 150 mL

¾ cup = 175 mL

1 cup = 250 mL

1 quart = 1 liter

1-½ quarts = 1.5 liters

1 ounce = 30 grams

2 ounces = 55 grams

3 ounces = 85 grams

4 ounces (¼ pound) = 115 grams

8 ounces (½ pound) = 225 grams

16 ounces (1 pound) = 455 grams

1 pound = ½ kilogram

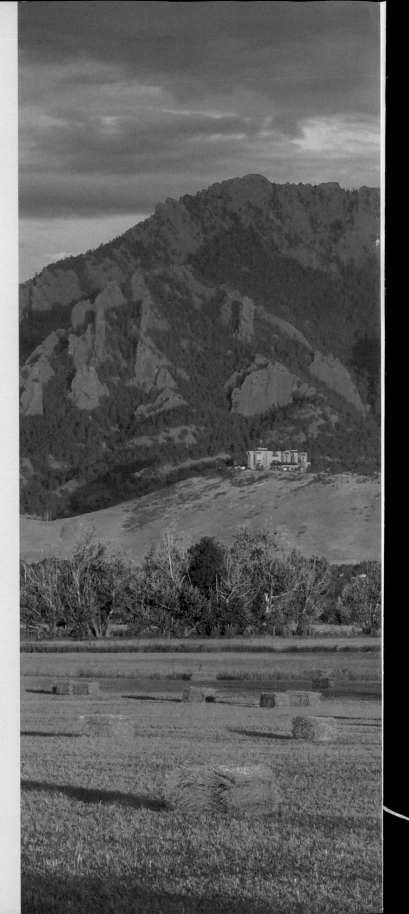

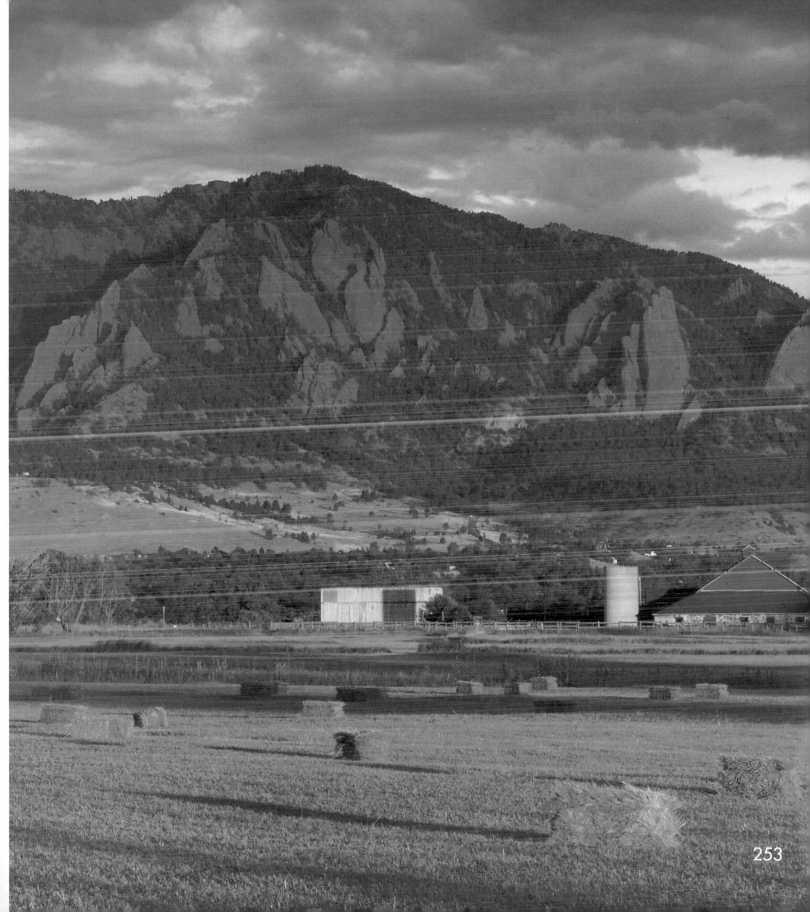

Glossary

14ers: A 14er (fourteener) is a mountain summit that rises above 14,000 feet from sea level. In Colorado, it is a "rite of passage" to climb your first 14er, since Colorado has the greatest number of 14ers in North America. Mount Elbert is the highest peak in Colorado at a height of 14,440 feet.

Agave or agave nectar (or syrup), is a sweet substance, similar in taste and texture as honey, just a little sweeter with a thinner consistency. Agave nectar comes from the Blue Agave plant. Agave nectar is made up primarily of glucose and fructose and is considered a lower glycemic sweetener. It is a great honey substitute for vegans, but due to the high fructose content, it may not be good for those with metabolic syndrome or diabetes.

Amaranth is a gluten-free seed grain raised around the world, primarily in Asia, North and South America. Amaranth is high in complete protein, especially the amino acid lysine. Amaranth has a nutty flavor and is great cooked up as a breakfast cereal or side dish and the flour makes a great addition to any gluten-free baking mix.

Antioxidants are chemical substances that help protect the body from the adverse effects of oxygen. But if oxygen is necessary for life, why do we need to be protected from it? While it is true that oxygen is an essential energy source for our cells, unstable oxygen can actually be toxic and damaging to our bodies. Unstable oxygen is what we have in free radicals. Free radicals are formed as a result of factors like excess exposure to the sun, cigarette smoke and air pollution, excess alcohol, and even x-rays. Free radicals can damage the body's cells and DNA, and interrupt the normal ability to reproduce healthy cells. This is what happens for example, with cancer and heart disease. Antioxidants fight back against free radical damage, which is why they are essential for almost everyone. We can find antioxidants within the body or we can find them in the foods we eat or supplements we take. Green tea is one example a beverage that contains naturally occurring antioxidants.

Arrowroot is a thickening agent and a great alternative to cornstarch for anyone who wants or needs to avoid corn products. Arrowroot comes from a plant indigenous to the West Indies, *Marantha arundinacea*. Two teaspoons of arrowroot can be substituted for one tablespoon of cornstarch. One teaspoon of arrowroot can be substituted for one tablespoon of flour. It is best to mix arrowroot first with cool liquids before adding it to hot liquids.

Burdock root has many nutrients like iron, inulin (a carbohydrate), and beneficial oils. Burdock may enhance the performance of many of the organs which purify the body and eliminate toxins or waste (like the kidneys, liver, colon, etc).

Cacao is part of the Theobroma genus. It is more commonly referred to as chocolate. Chocolate is made from the cacao seeds, which are either dried at low temperature (to be classified as raw) or roasted. Small pieces of roasted cacao beans are called cacao nibs. Cacao nibs taste a lot like roasted coffee beans, somewhat nutty and bitter. Cacao contains antioxidants, magnesium, and sulfur. It also contains phylethylamine, which may be responsible for the euphoria that some people feel after eating chocolate.

Carotenoids are a family of provitamin A compounds responsible for giving many fruits and vegetables their bright colors (especially red, yellow, and orange). Carotenoids are immune-supportive antioxidants that may play a role in helping to prevent certain cancers.

Curry is best classified as a variety of spices that often includes curry leaves, turmeric, coriander, cumin, and red pepper – but the combination of spices can vary considerably depending on the type of cuisine. Curry powder is available commercially, as is curry paste. The bright yellow color of curry powder is due to turmeric, which is known as a powerful anti-inflammatory agent. Curry and turmeric have been studied for their potential benefit against degenerative diseases including Alzheimer's.

Edamame is soybeans, still in their pods. They are usually boiled or steamed before eating and sprinkled lightly with sea salt. Edamame is found in most grocery stores and Asian markets in the frozen food section. It may also be found near the prepared food section, especially if the grocer offers sushi. It is very common in Asian cuisine.

Essential Fatty Acids (EFAs) are necessary fats that humans cannot synthesize, and must be obtained through diet. EFAs are long-chain polyunsaturated fatty acids derived from linolenic, linoleic, and oleic acids. EFAs support the cardiovascular, reproductive, immune, and nervous systems. The human body needs EFAs to manufacture and repair cell membranes, enabling the cells to obtain optimum nutrition and expel harmful waste products. EFA deficiency and Omega 6/3 imbalance is linked with serious health conditions, such as heart attacks, cancer, insulin resistance, asthma, lupus, schizophrenia, depression, postpartum depression, accelerated aging, stroke, obesity, diabetes, arthritis, ADHD, and Alzheimer's Disease, among others.

Flaxseed oil may be used as a dietary supplement. It has one of the highest, if not the highest, alpha-linolenic acid content of any plant oil. Flaxseed oil must be kept refrigerated as the oil itself is quite susceptible to rancidity.

Fair Trade (also spelled fair-trade) advocates fair wages to producers and growers of products (mostly in developing countries). It is a structured movement that works by helping communities and individuals work towards greater sustainability and self-sufficiency. Fair Trade strategies target exports from developing countries to developed countries. Coffee, chocolate, sugar, tea, and cotton are among some of the more common Fair Trade products. Fair Trade certification, which allows products to carry the "Fairtrade Certified" label claim, is overseen by FLO International and FLO-CERT.

Fiber is a type of carbohydrate that moves through the digestive tract basically unchanged. Fiber helps us feel more full and more satisfied because it slows digestion and absorption so that sugar (glucose) enters the bloodstream more slowly. There are two main types of fiber, soluble and insoluble. Soluble fiber dissolves in water and has a positive effect in the body including lowering bad cholesterol and blood sugar levels. Insoluble fiber cannot be dissolved in water and helps with regularity/elimination. Adults would do well to eat at least 28 grams of fiber daily.

Flavonoids are a class of compounds that are most commonly known for their antioxidant activity. Flavonoids and flavonols come from plants and have health modulating effects when consumed.

Free range is a marketing term used to describe a method of raising livestock where the animals are permitted to roam freely as opposed to being contained. It may also imply other meanings including grass fed, humanely raised, or pasture raised. It is assumed that free range meats and eggs come from animals allowed to graze on grasses, rather than corn fed.

Ghee is a clarified butter without any solid milk particles or water. Ghee is used in India and throughout South Asia in daily cooking. A good quality ghee adds a great aroma, flavor and taste to the food.

Gluten is a starchy wheat protein, made from the proteins gliadin and glutenin, present in many grass grains including wheat, rye, barley, kamut, and spelt. It is estimated that approximately 1% of the United States population has an adverse immune (autoimmune) response to gluten, labeled celiac disease. When individuals with celiac disease eat foods that contain gluten, damage can occur in the small intestine. This can then lead to malabsorption of essential vitamins, minerals, and other nutrients, which then can cause other health problems.

Glycemic Index (GI) is a ranking (0 to 100) of foods according to their effect on blood glucose levels. High GI foods (ranking of 70 and above) are quickly digested and can result in wacky blood sugar fluctuations. Low GI foods (55 and under) are digested and absorbed more slowly and have been shown to be beneficial to people with both type 1 and type 2 diabetes. Low GI foods also help with weight management and appetite control. Examples of low GI foods include dark green leafy vegetables (broccoli, cabbage, lettuce, kale), onions, carrots, peas, cherries, plums, grapefruit, peaches, apples, pears, coconut, grapes, berries, whole milk, yogurt, legumes, brown rice, wheat tortillas, buckwheat, new potatoes, sweet potatoes, whole grain pasta, rolled oats, oat bran, nuts, and seeds.

Greek-Style Yogurt is a thicker, creamier, richer style of yogurt that has higher protein content than most regular style yogurts.

Greens or Powdered Greens are generally a powdered form of phytonutrients made from foods like fruits, vegetables, seaweeds, herbs, and/or grasses. Nutritional information and taste can vary considerably between greens products. Look for greens that do not contain artificial sweeteners, colors, or flavoring agents.

High Fructose Corn Syrup (HFCS) is a sweetener to avoid. It is a highly refined sugar that the body doesn't metabolize very well. HFCS is added to a wide array of foods ranging from sweets to condiments. It has been linked to increased rates of obesity. HFCS is made by milling corn to produce corn starch, which is made into corn syrup, which is roughly total glucose, and then changing the glucose into fructose through an additional process. It is often added to foods you wouldn't suspect, so please read labels.

Medium Chain Triglycerides or MCTs, are (medium chain) fatty acids that are found in foods like coconut oil and palm kernel oil. Some research suggests that MCTs have a positive effect on metabolism and burning excess calories.

Mindful Eating is a bit like a meditation practice in that we focus our attention on the present experience, in this case, eating. Mindful eating means freeing ourselves from outside distractions while we are eating, including watching television, driving, working in front of the computer or other forms of multitasking. It means being conscious of the selection, portion, timing, and environment in which we eat. Mindful eating may have a positive impact on many aspects of physical, mental, and emotional health.

mix1 is an enhanced protein/antioxidant beverage that provides balanced nutrition in the form of carbohydrates, protein, healthy fat, fiber, and antioxidants. Check out www.mix1life.com for more information

Naturopathic Medicine is based on the belief that the human body has an innate healing ability. Naturopathic doctors (NDs) teach their patients to use diet, exercise, lifestyle changes and cutting edge natural therapies to enhance their bodies' ability to ward off and combat disease. NDs view the patient as a complex, interrelated system (a whole person), not as a clogged artery or a tumor. Naturopathic physicians craft comprehensive treatment plans that blend the best of modern medical science and traditional natural medical approaches to not only treat disease, but to also restore health. For more information, visit www.naturopathic.org.

Organic foods, according to the USDA, are described as: Organic meat, poultry, eggs and dairy products come from animals that are given no antibiotics or growth hormones. Organic food is produced without using most conventional pesticides, fertilizers made with synthetic ingredients or sewage sludge, bioengineering or ionizing radiation.

Phytonutrients are chemical-like compounds found in plants that have shown promise in disease prevention. They can be further classified into different antioxidant groupings including flavonoids, carotenoids, isoflavones, lignans, saponins, and indoles.

Polyphenols are chemical compounds found in certain foods that may be beneficial to our health. Polyphenols have antioxidant activity that may help reduce the risk of heart disease and certain cancers. Food sources include tea, red wine and grapes, berries, cocoa, walnuts, pomegranates, peanuts, prunes, raisins, blueberries, kale, strawberries, spinach, raspberries, Brussels sprouts, plums, broccoli, beets, oranges, red grapes, red bell peppers, cherries.

Probiotics are little living microorganisms that inhabit our intestines. Most probiotic activity takes place in the small intestine. People usually eat yogurt because they hear it is healthy for them – and those health benefits are generally attributed to probiotics. Probiotics are also called beneficial bacteria because they help restore intestinal balance and improve gastrointestinal (GI) conditions like constipation, diarrhea, colon cancer, inflammatory bowel diseases, gas and bloating, *Helicobacter pylori* infection (the main cause of gastric ulcers), lactose intolerance, allergies, obesity, and yeast infections. Examples of probiotics include *Lactobacillus acidophilus, Lactobacillus casei, Lactobacillus plantarum and Lactobacillus brevis,* and *Bifodobacterium.*

Protein Powder

Whey protein is typically available in three major types: concentrate, isolate, and hydrolysate. It is a very well digested protein. Whey protein concentrate contains a fairly low level of fat and cholesterol, lactose, carbohydrate, and can fluctuate considerably in protein content. Whey protein isolate has typically had the fat and lactose removed. Isolates have a higher percentage of protein by weight. Whey protein hydrolysates are the most easily absorbed and least allergenic varieties of whey protein. Both whey protein concentrate and isolate have a milky flavor, while the hydrolysate form has a more bitter taste.

Whey protein contains branched chain amino acids (BCAAs), which are used to build and fuel muscles. Whey protein contains amino acids like cysteine and glutamine, which can be used to synthesize glutathione in the body. Glutathione is a powerful antioxidant that may help protect against certain types of cancer.

Soy protein is a popular protein choice among vegans. Soy protein isolate comes from defatted soy flour which has had most of the non-protein components, fats and carbohydrates removed. It contains roughly 90% protein by weight. Because of this, it has a neutral flavor and will cause less flatulence due to bacterial fermentation. Soy protein concentrate preserves much of the fiber of the original soybean, and contains about 70% protein.

Both **whey and soy protein powders** are widely available at most grocery stores and natural food stores. Other forms of protein powder that are available but sometimes more difficult to find, include hemp protein, brown rice protein (and sprouted rice protein), pea protein, and egg white protein.

Quercetin is a flavonoid that has demonstrated anti-inflammatory, antihistamine, antioxidant, and antiviral activity in the body. Quercetin has also exhibited antitumor activity against several cancers. Quercetin is found naturally in onions, apples, citrus fruits, dark berries and cherries, olive oil, buckwheat, grapes, tea, beans, and red wine.

Quinoa is a higher protein "ancient" seed-grain, naturally gluten-free, and really not a grain or a seed, but rather a fruit. Quinoa grows three to six feet high and the seed-grains are in clusters at the end of the stalk. There is a natural, bitter saponin residue that coats the seeds so the quinoa needs to be well-rinsed prior to cooking. Quinoa (pronounced Keen-wah), is a relative of spinach and Swiss chard. It is a nutty seed-like "ancient grain" that is high in complete protein, magnesium, manganese, iron, tryptophan and fiber. Quinoa is a great choice for vegan vegetarians due to its unique complete protein and it is naturally gluten-free. We usually rinse quinoa two or three times to remove the soapy saponin residue that can coat the seed.

Ratatouille is a traditionally prepared French stew that usually consists of garlic, eggplant, onions, summer squash, tomatoes, and bell peppers.

Sustainability (or Sustainable Cuisine) is a social movement towards maintaining well-being of ourselves and the planet. From the foods we choose to the energy we use, we can take this movement and its positive momentum to shift our lives in a direction of greater good and conscious creativity. Sustainability begins first as an inside job and grows powerfully outward from there. In the way that we consciously choose to eat with mindfulness, to the type of vehicle we drive and size of houses we choose, sustainability begins with choosing.

Sucanat is a naturally produced, unrefined cane sugar. It tastes a little bit like brown sugar, but is more granular like raw sugar.

Tamari is Japanese soy sauce made using traditional brewing methods. It tastes basically the same as soy sauce. We always use San-J Organic Wheat-Free Reduced Sodium Tamari that is a certified gluten-free product.

Teff is a tiny little nutty grain that is high in protein, calcium, and iron. It is found in the form of flour or as a whole grain and is naturally gluten-free.

Tempeh is a soy food made from partially cooked and fermented soybeans. It has high protein content and can be marinated, stir fried, baked, or stewed.

Tofu, also known as bean curd, originated in China and is made by coagulating soy milk. Tofu is a decent source of protein, is high in iron, and usually a good source of magnesium and calcium, depending on how it was processed.

Trans Fats may occur naturally in meat and dairy products, but they are also produced during the process of hydrogenation of oils. Partially hydrogenated oils add shelf life to processed foods, but they also increase the risk for coronary heart disease and metabolic syndrome.

Tryptophan is an amino acid found in poultry, red meat, eggs, chocolate, oats, dates, mangoes, dried dates, milk, yogurt, cottage cheese, red fish, chickpeas, sunflower seeds, pumpkin seeds, sesame seeds, and peanuts. Tryptophan has been used as a sleep aid and as anti-depressant in mild depression and seasonal affective disorder.

Fit Kitchen Resources

We are often asked where to find and purchase some of our favorite foods, beverages, and dietary supplements. We've compiled a list for you here, which is not meant to be mutually exclusive, but rather give you a great place to start building your own Fit Kitchen.

Chicken and Vegetable Broths
Pacific Foods
9480 SW 97th Ave.
Tualatin, OR 97062
503-692-9666
Fax 503-692-9610
www.pacificfoods.com

Chips and Crackers
Mary's Gone Crackers
P.O. Box 965
Gridley, CA 95948
888-258-1250
Fax 530-846-5500
www.marysgonecrackers.com

Food Should Taste Good
PO Box 776
Needham Heights, MA 02494
www.foodshouldtastegood.com

Flours, Oats and Grains
Bob's Red Mill
13521 SE Pheasant Court
Milwaukie, Oregon 97222
800-349-2173
Fax 503-653-1339

Living Harvest
Living Harvest Foods, Inc.
P.O. Box 4407
Portland, OR 97208
888-690-3958
www.livingharvest.com

Arrowhead Mills
The Hain Celestial Group
4600 Sleepytime Dr.
Boulder, CO 80301
800-434-4246
www.arrowheadmills.com

Food Dehydrator
Excalibur Products
6083 Power Inn Road
Sacramento, CA 95824
800-875-4254
ww.excaliburdehydrator.com

Gluten-Free Bread and Pizza Crust
Udi's
101 East 70th Avenue
Denver CO, 80221
303-657-1600
Fax 303-657-1615
www.udisfood.com

Kinnikinnick Foods
877-503-4466
780-421-0456
www.kinnikinnick.com

Dad's Gluten Free Pizza
1867 N. Firebrick Drive
Kuna, ID 83634
www.glutenfreepizza.com

Greek-Style Yogurt
Oikos
Stonyfield Farm
10 Burton Drive
Londonberry, NH 03053
800-776-2697
www.stonyfield.com/oikos

Voskos
www.voskos.com

Greens
Nano-greens
112 N. Curry Street
Carson City, Nevada, 89703
877-464-6284
www.nano-greens.com

Healthy Frozen and Canned Foods
Amy's Kitchen, Inc.
PO Box 449
Petaluma, CA 94953
707.578.7270
www.amys.com

Cascadian Farms
Small Planet Foods
P.O. Box 9452
Minneapolis, MN 55440
800-624-4123
www.cascadianfarm.com

Muir Glen
Small Planet Foods
P.O. Box 9452
Minneapolis, MN 55440
800-624-4123
www.muirglen.com

Westbrae
The Hain Celestial Group, Inc.
4600 Sleepytime Dr.
Boulder, CO 80301
800-434-4246
www.westbrae.com

Nutritional Supplements

Nature's Code
800-367-9444
www.qvc.com/naturescode

Organic Dairy & Meat Products

Organic Valley Family of Farms
CROPP Cooperative
One Organic Way
LaFarge, WI 54639
888-444-6455
Fax 608-625-3025
www.organicvalley.coop
www.organicprairie.coop

Applegate Farms
750 Rt. 202 South, Suite 300
Bridgewater, NJ 08807-5530
866-587-5858
Fax 800-358-8289
www.applegatefarms.com

Niman Ranch
1600 Harbor Bay Parkway, Suite 250
Alameda, CA 94502
www.nimanranch.com

Laura's Lean Beef
1517 Bull Lea Road, Suite 210
Lexington, Kentucky 40511
859-299-7707
Fax 859-299-6822
www.laurasleanbeef.com

Organic and Biodynamic Wine

Cono Sur
Viña Cono Sur S.A.
Av. Nueva Tajamar 481 Torre Sur
Oficina 2101, Las Condes
Santiago, Chile
56-2-4765090
Fax56-2-2036732
www.conosur.com

Cooper Mountain Wine
9480 SW Grabhorn Rd
Beaverton, OR 97007
503-649-0027
ww.coopermountainwine.com
Fax 503-649-0702

Girasole Vineyards
7051 N. State Street
Redwood Valley CA 95470
707-485-0322
Fax 707 485 6704
www.girasolevineyards.com

The Organic Wine Company
www.theorganicwinecompany.com

Safe Seafood Sources

www.montereybayaquarium.org

Snacks

mix1 Nutritional Beverage
1965 North 57th Court, Suite 102
Boulder, CO 80301
www.mix1life.com

Soy Products (Tofu, Tempeh, Soymilk)

White Wave Foods
12002 Airport Way
Broomfield, CO 80021-2546
(303) 635-4000
www.whitewave.com

San-J International (wheat-free tamari)
2880 Sprouse Drive
Richmond, Virginia 23231
800-446-5500
Fax 804-226-8383
www.san-j.com

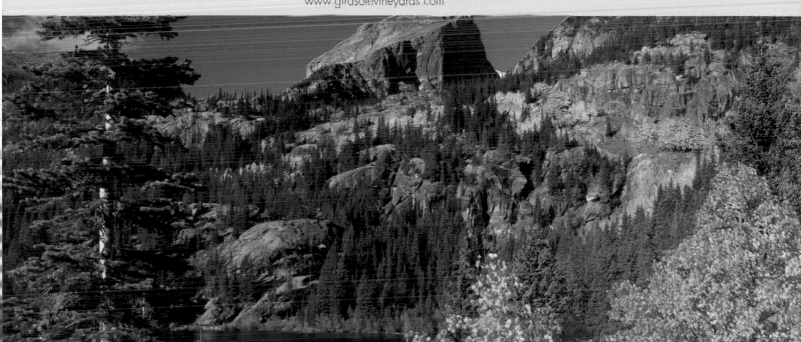

Index

263

Dr. James Rouse

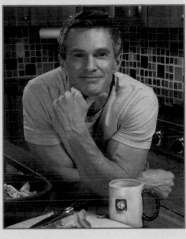

A naturopathic doctor, Ironman triathlete, QVC Network Wellness Doctor, entrepreneur, certified yoga instructor, wellness magazine founder, speaker, author, radio talk show host and television personality – Dr. James does it all. He talks with such enthusiasm and conviction about the wellness lifestyle, you come away feeling inspired to take better care of yourself – and to enjoy your life more.

James is best known for his highly engaging "Optimum Wellness" TV segments, which he hosts in major markets including Los Angeles, Seattle and Denver. These segments highlight all areas of a wellness lifestyle, balancing mind, body, and spirit.

His wellness knowledge and passion for helping others live life optimally also extends to creating healthy food products. Dr. James recently launched mix1, an all-natural nutritional beverage, blending antioxidant nutrients with a balance of carbohydrates and protein for pre- and post-workout and to support overall performance. He also serves as QVC's Wellness doctor.

When he's not flying across the country evangelizing about living well, he authors books including Grow Your Life from Average to Amazing; and Gaiam's Health Solutions for Stress Relief, Health Solutions for Sleep, Health Solutions for Weight Loss, and Health Solutions for Energy.

James loves endurance sports and anything involving exercise, especially cycling and telemark skiing.

Dr. Debra Rouse

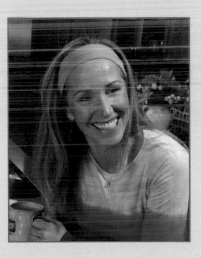

Dr. Debra Rouse is a naturopathic doctor with extensive clinical experience in nutrition, botanical medicine, women's and children's health, homeopathy, lifestyle medicine and physical conditioning.

She is the co-creator of the Optimum Wellness media program, which includes television, web and retail presence, and bimonthly magazine seen and read throughout Colorado, Southern California and the Northwest.

Debra is dedicated to educating and inspiring others to take charge of their health through community outreach seminars, articles, retreats, radio, and creating healthy recipes. Debra served as senior writer and editor for alternative and complementary medicine for Micromedex, a division of Thomson Healthcare, and continues freelance writing and editing. Her writing and recipes have been featured in such magazines as Delicious Living, Better Nutrition, Vegetarian Times, and Alternative Medicine.

Debra is a certified NIA instructor, has completed marathons, triathlons, including a half-Ironman triathlon, and loves cycling, tennis, skiing, snowshoeing, and hiking with the family.